CARING FOR MARIA

Bernard Heywood has had a varied career which includes teaching, travel, freelance journalism, posts with the British Hospitality Association and service in the army during the war. He has also had plays produced by professional actors and has written and published poems and articles. He is currently retired and living in Dorset, England.

Caring for Maria

An Experience of Successfully Coping with Alzheimer's Disease

BERNARD HEYWOOD

ELEMENT

Shaftesbury, Dorset ● Rockport, Massachusetts
Brisbane, Queensland

© Bernard Heywood 1994

Published in Great Britain in 1994 by
Element Books Ltd
Longmead, Shaftesbury, Dorset

Published in the USA in 1994 by
Element, Inc.
42 Broadway, Rockport, MA 01966

Published in Australia in 1994 by
Element Books Ltd
for Jacaranda Wiley Ltd
33 Park Road, Milton, Brisbane, 4064

Cover design by Max Fairbrother
Design by Roger Lightfoot
Typeset by Create Publishing Services Ltd., Bath
Printed and bound in Great Britain by
Redwood Books, Trowbridge, Wilts.

British Library Cataloguing in Publication
data available

Library of Congress Cataloging in Publication
data available

ISBN 1-85230-502-9

Contents

Dedication

This book is dedicated to all those who in greater or smaller ways helped me so splendidly to look after Maria; and to those who, subsequently, with their encouragement or comments, moved me to start and then complete the book. I am very grateful to all of them.

It is also dedicated to all those who suffer from Alzheimer's disease or other forms of dementia, and to those who have the hard task of looking after them, privately or professionally. They have my empathy and best wishes.

I would also like to record my thanks to those who, at various stages, helped with the typing of the manuscript; to the many charities and individuals who so generously helped with the funding of the nurses; to Julia McCutchen of Element Books for the interest she showed in the original manuscript and the help that she gave; and, finally, to Barbara Horn for her very considerable expertise and help in editing and cutting the original mansucript to its present length.

Then, not to be forgotten is Maria herself. This book is also especially dedicated to her at her best and bravest. And I am sure that, in whatever way is now appropriate for her, she joins with me in my expressions of gratitude.

Prologue

This story is entirely true except that all the names of those mentioned in it, other than my own, are not their real names. The place names are true.

For nearly ten years I looked after Maria, an elderly lady who had Alzheimer's disease. Maria had been a close friend, whom my wife and I had known in London for many years, and when, on my retirement in 1971 we came to live in a small seaside village, Maria came with us. We moved to a complex of sheltered housing for the elderly run by a housing association, with a resident warden, where we shared a unit; my wife and I lived in a flat on the ground floor, and Maria lived in one immediately above. Her age at the time was 69, and mine was 65.

It was shortly after my wife died in 1977 that my years of caring for Maria began. They covered the beginning of Maria's Alzheimer's (though it was not recognized at the time), its build-up and its moderate and severe stages until she died in 1987. My commitment to Maria was comparatively limited at first but grew with her increasing deterioration until I was a full-time carer.

During this time I kept detailed diaries. It was a practice that I had started when my wife died. The entries were in the form of letters to her, and I found writing them therapeutic. They were also useful in stimulating thought and clarifying problems, and 'letting off steam'; and they were, of course, a record of events. I have used them as the basis of this book, summarizing, explaining and commenting on the events they describe, as well as including extracts just as they were written.

After Maria's death I was asked to give some talks about my

experience of caring to local carers' groups, who then encouraged me to write this book, which, I was assured, could not only be of value to other personal and professional carers, but also, because of its human story, interest a wider public. I was further persuaded by the thought that if the book could help other people, it would have the added merit of bringing some good out of the evil of Maria's affliction.

The book is in no sense a technical treatise. It is simply a detailed factual account of what Alzheimer's meant in all its day-to-day front-line detail for a particular sufferer and carer. It is, however, more than just a specific Alzheimer's story. It is as much a story of caring as of Alzheimer's itself. Also, other ailments from which Maria suffered intrude into the Alzheimer's picture, but they were so much a part of the situation that they could not be ignored.

No two cases of any disease run the same course. The details of individual sufferers and carers vary. However, basic similarities are generally constant and, in so far as its Alzheimer's element is concerned, this case is characteristic of what the disease can mean for both sufferer and carer, though there is one special feature. Maria was of German birth and gradually lost her ability to speak and, later to understand, English. Ultimately she spoke only German, so that communication was very difficult, for my German was at first non-existent, and though I took some lessons, it never became competent. While this language difficulty led to a special problem of communication, which was at times very distressing for us, it was not entirely abnormal. Difficulty of communication is, in varying measure, a common aspect of the disease, and the mental confusion and other symptoms are present in all cases.

Most of us are sometimes critical of others, even of those who are close to us, and I had been critical of Maria on various occasions before she had Alzheimer's. If the diaries seem critical of her behaviour at times, such criticism was only an instant and temporary reaction. That soon passed, for behind it was the realization that she was ill and suffering. And if the extracts from the diaries or my interpolations appear almost flippant at times, no one should imagine that the matter was, or is now, being treated lightly. I cared greatly about what was happening to Maria, but if something is odd or laughable, it is still that even if it is also sad or tragic, and it does no one any good to pretend otherwise. Humour can be remedial; and if in some other life Maria has subsequently been able to see the past, I can certainly imagine her exclaiming, '*Du lieber Gott, Ich muss lachen*' (Dear God, I must laugh) at some of the things that happened.

Why did I take so much trouble to look after Maria? Why didn't I opt out at some stage when I could have done so 'with honour'? It is not always easy to understand *exactly* why we do certain things, but over the years I had seen Maria fighting a largely losing battle against the circumstances of her life, and doing so with great courage; she was in her way a remarkable person with many fine qualities. She was also a good friend – *not* anything more – and I cared about what happened to her. I had always felt that she had deserved better of the world than she had received since I knew her, and that she certainly did not merit being discarded on some scrap heap.

It was, in short, an assignment, which it would have been shameful to ignore, although I did not consciously think of it as such at the start, nor choose it; rather, it evolved. I certainly did not look after Maria because I needed something to occupy my time. Since my retirement, even during the period when my wife had been a partial invalid requiring a measure of attention, I had been active in many ways. Then, after my wife died and I had worked through the time of immediate bereavement (during which Maria had been a real help to me), there was virtually no limit to the activities that beckoned. But if I had ignored Maria, particularly as I had no urgent conflicting obligations, I am sure I would have felt disgusted with myself. I would have been no less disgusted if I had later turned my back on her at any stage, for she showed at times great spirit in trying to rally herself against her affliction.

Various sources of inspiration or rationalizing notions (some sublime, some more mundane) bolstered me at times, but there was one that was especially important. I believe (as many others do) that there are operating in the world a good originating force, which can conveniently be called 'God', and a contrary evil force, which can conveniently be called 'the devil'. I also believe that illness for its own sake is *not* the will of the good force, of God, but is basically the evil force, the devil, causing in a vast variety of ways the disorders that damage the human body and psyche. I further believe that for some reason not apparent to our human intelligence, or at any rate not to mine, life is a contest between good and evil, and that we are fulfilling our proper destiny when we are fighting, or at least living, on the side of obvious good against obvious evil.

As Maria's dementia built up, I came to regard it more and more as the work of the evil force, the devil; and I looked upon my caring for her as being a small contribution to the overall fight of good against evil. It thus became in part something of a personal contest between me and the devil. Rationalizing it as such was both an added reason for carrying out my task and a help in doing so.

Whenever I succeeded in making Maria's life somewhat happier or kept my temper when her demented behaviour exasperated me, I could then imagine that I was landing a sharp blow (preferably in some sensitive spot) on the devil and frustrating his evil ploy. On such occasions I would sometimes picture him sulking and skulking in a corner, or when something had gone particularly well, I might visualize him (in the guise of the old designer devil) running away with his horns crumpled, his tail between his legs and his pitchfork bent double; and perhaps I would imagine, or even actually mutter, a cry of 'Ha! Ha!' after his departing form. I fully accept that this may, in whole or in part, seem nonsensical or farfetched to some people, but it was a significant help to me; and when in the diaries there are occasional references to the devil, this is how they should be understood.

Maria

Maria was a handsome woman of average height, sturdy rather than slim. Even at the age of 85, and despite her hard life, her face was virtually unlined and her dark auburn hair showed scarcely a trace of grey. She had a splendid smile, but when the mood was on her, she could look truly grim. Indeed, such were the paradoxes in this colourful and many-sided personality that I sometimes felt that Maria was two people. She had a charisma, something more than mere charm, which could enchant and hold both women and men, yet she could be domineering and her presence almost disturbing. Good-natured, polite and ready to help others, Maria would perform acts of kindness beyond the conventional, but she could also be self-centred, critical and rude. She was ready to praise people when there was a reason, but she could also be too easily, and often wrongly, suspicious and accusatory. Naturally outgoing and lively, she could also be withdrawn and introspective.

Born in 1902, Maria came from a family of high social standing, which had lived very comfortably on a large estate in East Prussia until the First World War. Following the war, Maria married and had two sons. The family suffered further hardships in the Second World War, during which Maria was associated with an anti-Hitler resistance movement in Berlin. Some time after the end of the war Maria was divorced and become disillusioned with contemporary Germany; and in 1949 she came to England, a country for which she had a great admiration as it then was. However, and this is only speculation, I believe that her move must have been prompted by something more traumatic, perhaps stemming from a war-time experience, for although she was apt to be impulsive, she was not prone to run away from things.

Maria was never prepared to talk about her past in any detail, so it was largely unknown to me, but I do know that her separation from her sons, of whom she was, and remained, very fond, was a source of real sorrow to her. She talked about them regularly and proudly, and she undoubtedly missed them. This seemed to increase as her Alzheimer's developed, and she would sometimes murmur sadly to herself, '*Meine Kinder*' (my children). As well as her sons, Maria had two sisters, a brother and various nieces and nephews in Germany. She kept in touch with them through fairly regular correspondence and occasional visits.

Maria came to England on a domestic permit, which was the only employment open to her as a non-specialist alien. Whatever the reason for her move, I have always regarded it as a remarkably courageous act. There she was, a cultured, intelligent, lively woman of high social standing, aged nearly 50, coming to work as a domestic servant in a country whose language she barely spoke, in which she knew no one, and which had recently been an enemy. It could perhaps have been regarded as foolhardy, but it certainly showed spirit.

Her first jobs were as cook-housekeeper in and near London, and during this time she experienced some unpleasantness. She then worked as a ward maid in a London hospital and as a chambermaid in a large London hotel, the latter post enabling her to 'live out' in a small bed-sitting room. Throughout this time Maria studied English, visited many of London's museums, galleries, churches and other places of interest, and went swimming regularly.

My wife and I got to know Maria in 1950 or 1951, when she joined a group that met in our flat. After a while I obtained permission for her to help in the office of an organization connected with European refugees with which I was associated. Shortly after this Maria became a British citizen, which meant that she could take up any work. She took courses in copy-typing, dressmaking and facial massage, and managed to support herself from these sources on a self-employed basis. She tried hard to find steadier employment, but although her spoken and written English were by now adequate, her age, national origin and relative lack of qualifications were against her, and her efforts came to nothing. I saw this for myself, and admiring her spirit and qualities, I tried to help her.

Throughout the years in London Maria continued to develop her interests in the city, and became particularly well informed on Westminster Abbey and the Tower of London. She taught herself a surprising amount about certain periods of English history, particularly the Tudors and the Stuarts, and compiled two splendid scrapbooks on them. She also meditated a great deal, and in her late fifties became a Roman Catholic.

When she became eligible for her state pension, Maria added painting to her other activities. She worked in oils, watercolours, crayon and charcoal. Over the years she turned out many excellent paintings, particularly, though not exclusively, of flowers. There were also a number of unusual Madonnas and Child. When we came to live near the sea, Maria was able to pursue her love of nature as well as maintaining her other interests. She walked a lot and tried to keep as fit as the advancing years and her ailments would allow. She explored the neighbouring countryside, learned about local bird life, kept up her swimming and developed the small garden that we shared. She also found a new interest: mountaineering. From the books that she studied, she knew who had climbed what and when; and if you had dropped her in the Western Cwm, she would have known how to climb to the top of Everest by the South Col route.

These latter years before Alzheimer's took over were perhaps the happiest time of Maria's life in England, for despite all the interests of London, she had had a very hard struggle there, suffering many disappointments in the face of her considerable efforts to make a success of her life. I saw all of it and never ceased to admire her courage, determination and unfailing lack of bitterness.

Alzheimer's disease is a physical ailment that causes a progressive decline in the ability to remember, to learn, to think and to reason. Although a great deal of research is being done on it and various possibilities are being investigated, its basic cause is not yet known, but it is associated with abnormal functions of the brain cells, which suffer characteristic changes. It can affect some younger people, but the vast majority of sufferers are older people and there is an increased risk of developing it with increasing age.

The First Period

1. *December 1977 to 14 April 1982*

In the late 1970s Maria, who was then in her own late seventies, began to have increasing physical problems. Those that she had previously had became more marked, including arthritis in the spine and left knee, which had virtually no cartilage left. Her heart trouble worsened, and she had stomach pains from time to time. Despite these various pains, Maria was reluctant to take painkillers, which, she said, 'don't cure you, they merely hide what's wrong'. She also suffered from headaches and dizziness, and had occasional blackouts and minor falls; and she would say such things as 'My brain seems empty', 'My legs won't obey me'. In the past when she had wanted something, she would usually come downstairs and knock on my door. Now, and increasingly as her physical health deteriorated, she would thump on her floor to call me upstairs.

In addition to these physical ailments Maria started to seem a bit odd: forgetful and confused about things that had hitherto been no problem. She exhibited a growing security complex, with unrealistic suspicions that people were against her or deceiving her, which led her to change the lock on her door quite often and to make unjustified accusations. The latter had happened before, but to a very much more limited extent and with far less emphasis. It was also about now that Maria started to speak German occasionally instead of English.

All this could be trying for both Maria and me, but I thought it was just a routine aspect of old age. The idea of dementia or Alzheimer's (of which I'd never heard) did not occur to me, for Maria's oddities were spasmodic rather than regular and, by and large, she carried on with her normal activities. But mentally she was not what she used to be, and as I look back I realize that dementia was building up.

The earliest sign of what was to come that I can remember was an incident that puzzled me at the time, but which in hindsight seems like incipient Alzheimer's. Maria accused a friend, Miss Barrett, of failing to repay some money. Maria had owed Miss Barrett a small sum and claimed that, not having the exact amount, she had given her £5 and was due the change. She was emphatic, almost aggressive, that this was the case. Miss Barrett, however, was equally certain that she had been paid the correct amount and therefore did not owe Maria any money. Although I supported Maria, I had a feeling that she might have had a lapse of memory, and I was surprised at her uncompromising attitude. In the event Miss Barrett paid the required sum, but the friendship came to an end.

Beginning in December 1977 I began to notice over (rather surprisingly) a relatively short period of time most of the features that subsequently occurred during the entire building-up process. I noted in my diary for the first time Maria's various ailments, her cancellation of appointments, my keeping her company more often than previously, my shopping and going to the library for her, and my growing feeling that I might have a duty to help her. There are also references, as there would be for the rest of her life, to her courage and spirit, though even then she would sometimes shake her head despondently and say: 'What can I do?' She continued to be generous and helpful to me from time to time, but this was frequently and increasingly interspersed with accusations that I stole from her.

The first such accusation came in January 1978. When I told Maria she was wrong, she said that I was evil and made her sick. Yet the next day she was quite 'sane' again. Such accusations followed by normal behaviour were to become a constant pattern.

In May Maria began to visit Dr Brown (a consultant physician) about her general health. He took a great deal of trouble over her, despite her cancellations of many appointments and, later, her difficulty in communicating. In addition to her physical ailments, he noted that she was somewhat paranoid about me, accusing me of theft, 'womanizing' and of generally being a bad character – 'a

lecherous crook', as he colourfully described it. I knew this, for
Maria said as much to me on occasion, but mainly I shrugged it off. I
knew it wasn't true, and I remembered being told that some elderly
people often 'take it out' on those who help them. It was not until
April 1982 that he felt sure that Maria had some form of dementia.

Early in 1979 I felt for the first time that to look after Maria might
be an intended job for me. Although at this time and for the next
couple of years she was still able to do many ordinary things for
herself, including going for walks, cooking and traveling to nearby
towns, and even to London and Germany, these 'good' periods were
becoming more and more offset by confusion, suspicion and
language problems. Her visits to Dr Brown became more difficult:
she was not able to explain things clearly to him, and she mis-
understood what he said. Maria was not unaware of these problems,
commenting 'I've got no more strength to fight even if I knew what
to fight against' and 'I'm like a machine that doesn't work'. She
would get very depressed, and I was sure that she cried when she was
alone. At one point I had some pain myself, which made me think
how brave she was with hers, which was far worse. I also realized,
later if not then, that carers can have their own troubles in addition
to those related to their caring and those of the people for whom
they are caring.

Sometimes I found it hard to contain myself at her behaviour, and
as time went on I often questioned whether I was doing right in
trying to help her in the way that I did, as the extracts from my diary
show.

9 December 1981   About 6.30am Maria thumped to say – can it
be possible that this goes on for ever? – that she can't go to Dr
Brown today. She's got such pain all over, she was almost in tears.
And though I shouldn't think of it and must carry on, how awful
for me: more cancellations, more apologies, more bewilderment,
more depression, more uncertainty about the future. Phoned to
cancel the car [we regularly used the local taxi, driven by Mr or
Mrs Mason] and then Dr Brown. He was so understanding.

The TV repairman came to check Maria's set. He had to take it away; she wondered if it would be returned without some part having been stolen!

12 December   Maria got into one of her awkward moods including more complaints about her TV (now back in one piece). I can't see anything wrong, but she has developed a sort of obsession about it. She seems to think everybody's doing her down, and is determined to take it out on someone or something – me or the television for instance . . .

How ought I to handle her and (to put it compassionately) her troubled mind? Agree with her however wrong she may be? Or contest it? Contesting does no good, because she just thinks I'm stupid, whereas to agree with her can be unfair to the facts or to other people . . . Ultimately she was happy that the TV was all right, but without any rebuttal of her past observations. One just has to treat her patiently as a sick person.

13 December   This afternoon Maria thumped to show me rain dripping on to her sitting-room floor through a hole at the top of the windowsill. She was also agitated about cold air coming in. I had to stuff something in the hole. Sat with her from 4.00 to 6.30, but after I came down, she thumped again wanting an antacid for her stomach. Is somebody sticking pins into an image of her, not to mention of me?

16 December   Went to watch TV with Maria. I ought to be doing something more productive . . . If only there was someone else to keep her company or she was still well enough to amuse herself. But what's the good of saying 'If only'? Absolutely none. There are times when I could almost scream at the things that I'm prevented from doing.

19 December   Went up to be with Maria for two and a half hours. She needs someone on to whom she can unload her complaints and to watch things with her. Almost frighteningly, it becomes more demanding. Apart from forty-five minutes, I've been doing something for her for all day from 7.00am to 6.00pm.

21 December   Frances [a friend with whom she had often gone walks in the past] came for coffee with Maria. Maria was in as good form personally and (apparently) physically as for some time … It would be splendid if she could stay like she is today and do more painting or things on her own.

26 December   No sign of Maria till she thumped at 2.25pm. She wants to continue in bed because of spinal pain. And – oh dear – she wants to cancel Dr Brown's appointment on Wednesday. These instant reactions of hers make for great confusion.

28 December   Maria thought someone rang her bell at 8.00am and wondered if it was me. It wasn't; she must have heard something else … She's not well and has not been able to get out for four or five days.

9 January 1982   Coffee with Maria and the usual 'argument' about her maintaining that she had given me something which she hadn't, but no hard feelings! She thumped to offer me hot ham with mushrooms and potatoes for lunch.

13 January   Maria surfaced early to say that she had a bad headache and would I cancel the optician's appointment for this pm. I'll leave it till midday, but if I do it will be the sixth cancellation out of nine recent appointments. Later she was not much better, so I cancelled.

14 January   Maria – surprise, surprise – having a good day, and we walked along the beach. I then had coffee with her and listened to her talking about the past. She was in good form. Her variability is extraordinary.

30 January   Maria has suddenly got a wrong idea about some pills that I'd got permission for her to import from the Continent. I've kept the relevant letters, and she has concluded from this that the tablets have come and that I've kept them for myself. She can get things so wrong.

February was a reasonably good month for Maria, though it had its ups and downs. Chief amongst its downs were a spell of flu, the removal of her last tooth and trouble with her dentures, and spells when the cold weather made bed the best place for her. There were, too, various disturbances and confusions, such as a new curtain rod of hers that didn't work properly, and invasions of workmen to insulate the flat and repair a window. Her difficulties over understanding things continued. She was again convinced her doorbell had been rung, this time in the middle of the night; this was almost certainly imaginary.

Nevertheless, there were definitely more pluses than of late. She was for the most part reasonably cheerful; she had an excellent visit to Dr Brown, was able to go to church on her own, was pleased to find that she'd lost some weight and could get into a particular skirt again, and had more walks than recently. She gave me useful advice about rearranging a room and cooked occasional meals for me; she had great pleasure in watching the birds and doing chores around her flat.

My caring involvement, for it was now there in a relatively limited way, though not really thought of as such, was made easier by these pluses, augmented by the absence of any accusations; and it was a tonic just to see her in any sort of continuing good form. My involvement, though, was always there – constant shopping and writing letters for her; arranging activities; helping her with walks when she was not so well; explaining things to her and to various workmen on her behalf. Overall, I always felt that I had to keep my eyes open and be ready to step in to help her. Nevertheless, I decided that I could go away for a week to visit my granddaughter and her family, particularly as Frances and Edith Bailey [another neighbour] would keep an eye on Maria, who was not yet at an advanced state of deterioration or permanent disability and could manage by herself up to a point.

3 March   Maria seemed remarkably cheerful. She'd been to Dr Brown and managed to go on her own to Salisbury and Dorchester … We chatted quite a while, mostly in English. And she made me coffee. It was all very congenial.

There were times like this when she had spells of talking English better, so that communication and all that went with it was naturally easier.

6 March   Maria thumped to say that she wouldn't be well enough to have Frances to coffee as arranged, so I cancelled her. Then she thumped to say she was now better, so I uncancelled!

11 March   Maria thumped just before breakfast to say that her kitchen wall heater wasn't working. I went up, pulled the string and it worked at once! She hadn't pulled hard enough!

The failures, uncertainties, mistakes, confusions, misunderstandings and suspicions that now began to crop up were a great contrast to the way that she had been before. Some of them may seem trivial, and her physical ailments may have been a partial cause, but now, as I look back, I can see them as definite indications of her early and developing Alzheimer's.

12 March   Walked to the seafront with Maria, which, apart from a strong wind, was pleasant with the sun. She managed surprisingly well considering she couldn't really walk yesterday.

14 March   Maria's in a very depressed state – tired and wanting, but unable, to do housework. It's impossible to do much to cheer her and I feel inadequate.

16 March   We talked – or rather Maria did – about her pains, and she said she'd have to cancel her appointment at the bank tomorrow. She was to discuss her will. However, on my return from shopping, she asked me to remind her to phone the bank tomorrow morning to confirm that she'd be going. One never knows!

17 March   She's now cancelled the bank appointment once more, as she is 'too ill', so I've revised the car arrangements for the third time.

19 March   I started to prepare notes about what I do for Maria, so that someone may be able to help her if I die first (unlikely).

22 March   There is a catalogue of things that want doing in connection with Maria and much else is looming. I think I must find a remote cave! But then it'd probably have a leak in the roof and some other cave dweller would want me to collect sticks ...

Back from Bridport, I visited Maria. Her capacity for not understanding what one is trying to say or to make plain what she means is getting almost frightening. Endless patience is required. I feel slightly ragged and have a headache.

24 March   I felt heavy-hearted about Maria. It's not nice to see and to feel for a lioness in winter who is deteriorating, yet who is still trying to fight and keep cheerful. It must be even less nice for her. The Lord loveth whom he chasteneth says the Psalms and I'm prepared to accept the truth of that up to a point; but I pray that she has the perpetual strength and comfort to endure and to apprehend the grace and growth that I am sure is inherent in her trials.

30 March   Maria thumped. She had pains in her heart. I got her to go to bed and, after drinking some wine, she seemed to improve, but she wants me to phone Dr Brown tomorrow to ask him what she should do. She puts it down to the cold weather, but I'm inclined to feel that it may be some kind of neurosis. But how can I tell and what can I do?

After we had some more wine, she said she'd keep to her bed and try to sleep. I stayed around; I certainly help with just doing that and with listening to her talk, and with having chocolate and biscuits available when she suddenly wants them as she often does. But I don't know what I'd do if she had some sort of major collapse.

31 March   Heard Maria moving at 6.30am so went up. Pain in back, arms and legs, but she slept all night and there was no further reference to her heart. She still wants me to phone Dr Brown, which is the sort of thing I hate doing – bothering people. Is it a weakness? I phoned and am waiting for him to phone back. But Maria, who has just thumped, now seems much better, so perhaps the call was unnecessary. This is typical Maria country. She never used to be so changeable.

Well, the doctor phoned at 7.00 pm – very kind after a hard day. He didn't think her pains were cardiac, and told me to reassure her. Not necessary to spend a long time in bed, but a glass of wine or whisky is excellent. She was pleased he'd phoned and glad of the advice, though she's sure it was to do with her heart.

4 April After breakfast I was getting down to doing more notes about Maria for my will, when she thumped. She was very depressed with her pain and could hardly move. She was depressed with everything. If only she could die, she'd be so pleased. We just don't know what to do. And I'm useless at helping her fundamentally. Not that she is always easy to help.

6 April I went up to watch a film on TV with Maria. However, she had to turn it off at the end as she didn't like the violence. Earlier she had suddenly become annoyed and anxious about the dust and had gone round the room dusting while the film was still on. I'm so sorry for her, but why must she let housework add to her troubles and pain? If you try to rationalize things, she just asks you not to argue. She then offered me coffee.

7 April Wrote a thank-you card for Maria to the Women's Fellowship, who had sent her a card. Though she can't now write English properly, she still has a right touch of expression for such things. She also took great trouble to choose a nice card from her collection. What a waste of her potential her life seems to have been, not that I know all that is involved or what is ultimately what. I so often feel that she should have been something like Queen of Liechtenstein instead of – as when I first knew her – scrubbing floors in hospitals and being exploited as a domestic servant, and then searching and searching for something fulfilling, but never finding it, and now ending up ill, crippled, poor and going out of her mind(?) despite all her efforts and courage and hope and trust and indomitable spirit. There has been such a waste of human material, and so much personal suffering beyond what seems to be merited. I say that with respect, and acknowledging – to God – that I may be wrong.

13 April Returned [from a short trip] to find that Maria had had a rotten time with pain and inability to walk. She'd managed to get down the stairs once to water some plants, but had had great difficulty in getting up again. Otherwise she spent most of the five days I was away in bed. Frances and Edith did some shopping for her. Her bad condition seems really prolonged at present. I'm worried, not only for her, but also at my increasing and increasingly hopeless and unavailing (it seems) commitment.

14 April Maria called me up to open a bottle of wine, just not knowing what to do with her head. 'I can't read. I can't watch television. I can't stay in the sitting-room because I get short of air. What can I do?' Yes, what can she do, other than keep seeing doctors and asking for more pills, which she won't do? She ought to tackle Dr Brown again, and she ought to keep appointments, or am I wrong? I'm just as restless and bewildered as she is.

The situation can induce in carers a sense of inadequacy, and a carer can, as it were, assimilate some of the restlessness and bewilderment of the sufferer, though their causes may be different.

2. 15 April 1982
to 10 March 1983

During the next few months I had a great deal of correspondence with Dr Brown about Maria's condition, especially her physical ailments. These weren't all in evidence all the time, but they were sufficiently regular to justify the correspondence. She suffered particularly from dizziness and swaying; constant headache and eye pain; some difficulty in keeping down food and little appetite; sweating at times, perhaps because of her many pains; swollen stomach and legs; pain in her knee, which often made walking difficult; and bad arthritis – she said it felt sometimes 'as if my spine is broken in half'. She would also comment 'I sway like a drunkard', 'I sit; and I can't even think', 'I can't understand it. There seems to be nothing I can do.' ... It was during the forthcoming weeks that Dr Brown suspected that Maria had Alzheimer's or some form of dementia.

> *15 April* 1982 Maria is terribly down, hardly able to walk, getting bad headaches and arthritis pain, and she can't eat. She wanted to have a bath, but she can't manage it; she can't risk going downstairs in case she can't get back; she can't do any housework. All of this adds to her depression. She repeatedly says, with her head in her hands, 'It's dreadful. What can I do?' It requires great patience not to be sharp with her, and great effort not to be flattened by her depression ... I must stay around as some sort of company for her.

One of the rationalizations (in addition to my contest with the devil) that I developed to help me to cope was to regard myself as akin to a prisoner of war who had to adjust until 'hostilities' ended. Another was to try to be a 'thoroughly professional amateur' as a carer. (Others will be mentioned as they occur.) I feel it is very important for carers to find as many such ways of their own as they can to help them cope.

17 April   Maria thumped and, blow me down, after struggling through some housework, she caught her foot in a chair and fell against the wardrobe with the chair on top of her. She seems to have bruised her wrist and perhaps her back.

21 April   Maria surfaced while I was eating my breakfast to ask if I had her rent book. If she can't find anything, she immediately assumes that it's something to do with me. But it's good that she feels up to tackling her rent.

29 April   Maria has just thumped to say that she can't find the key to her wardrobe, in which she keeps her money. This means that she can't go to the bank, as we had arranged, until she finds it. And she feels sick. Dear, oh dear! How it does go on! ... However, she seems to be sure that the key is in the flat, so she isn't imagining that I have taken it. She said that I ought to have a spare key for her wardrobe, and when I replied that I'd never had one, she said: 'Of course you had – you're a liar. I know because of what I found taken out of it after I'd been to Germany once.' The old crazy story.

Just as I wrote that, she thumped to tell me that she'd found the wardrobe key (what a saga!) in her bedclothes. I'd expected it to be there, amongst other possibilities, but I hadn't pressed the point, because she said that she'd looked everywhere. This has been yet another exercise for me in trusting and in not panicking.

1 May   Maria thumped when I was in the middle of my bath and became almost angry because I hadn't gone running upstairs.

She can get almost hysterical at times when I fail to go up in time to see something she wants me to see.

25 May   Maria is not very well and has confirmed cancelling an appointment with Dr Brown. I just don't know how justified such a decision is on purely physical grounds, but it's absolutely no way to get well or to find out what's what. She's so like a poor rat in a trap dashing about from one hope of escape to another, wondering what medicine she might take or what she can do to improve things; and in trying to cope and to help her I'm caught in her trap of confusion. There's really no one to help me except Dr Brown – and, of course, God. But I don't seem to be able to get through to him very well, and I've no idea what he's really doing or what he means me, or her, to do, except to keep on trying – flying, as it were, in a fog by radar.

4 June   Despite it being misty, Maria went into the sea. I stayed within reach, admiring her spirit. It was indeed a splendid and encouraging exercise of considerable value to her, both physically and psychologically.

9 June   Maria actually kept an appointment with Dr Brown, and both he and his wife were delighted with a lamp fitting that she'd bought for their daughter.

10 June   Maria enjoyed going into the sea although the weather wasn't too warm. She's very forgetful when she's 'not herself', and today she forgot to take down her sweater, and then she left her towel behind.

17 June   We had a very successful ten-hour trip, which took in Gloucester and its cathedral. On return, we had a drink with Edith Bailey and the trip organizer. Maria enjoyed it very much and she seemed, with the aid of occasional pills and resting off and on, to have managed it physically.

19 June   Maria went shopping and, lo and behold, when she came back, she found (or thought she found?) that her door was not locked. She immediately said that I'd been in her flat, 'like you've been before'. Oh dear, oh dear. I suppose she didn't lock the door properly. But it is distressing that she immediately assumes that I'm to blame. It's also stupid ...

Maria is convinced that I did another of a series of 'break-ins'. She says that she has a long list of all that I've taken, that this time she'll 'go to law'; that she's spent a fortune on new locks and keys but that I get copies of all of them; that I'm evil and that it's a sickness. Also she'll write to Dr Brown to tell him she can't see him any more as she can't take any more help from me (i.e., towards taxi fares). It's terribly distressing for her, because she sincerely believes it all. It is no less distressing for me, because she is totally wrong and I don't know what to do about it; while if I left, she'd be destitute of the help that she needs. Why should it suddenly happen just when things were looking hopeful?

I decided to go for a long walk. It was pleasant apart from this awful problem. I feel so much for her, and I realize how this hallucination must hurt and bedevil (literally) her and her life. But it's so wrong, and seems impossible to deal with. On return I wrote a note to her, trying to suggest what might ameliorate the situation for her, though I can't go so far as to say I'm guilty when I'm not; it would, I think, exacerbate the situation ... She thumped to ask if I wanted to go up and look at the news! I said I would. She added: 'I won't talk much.' I suppose she was referring to my note? What a human comedy (or tragedy) it is.

21 June   Maria wanted to know if she should tear the counterfoils off postal orders. This is an example of her fallibility. I told her about it yesterday, and several times in the past, but she doesn't remember anything. It's in such ways, amongst others, that my availability is a positive help to her.

23 June   As I was about to go to bed, Maria thumped. Haltingly, for communication in English seems to get progressively more difficult, she talked about Spanish history. I don't know why she got on to this, but she still seems to talk sense in such matters.

8 July   C.D. came to see me, and Maria, on her own initiative, brought us coffee at just the right moment . . . I spent two hours with her while she struggled to translate for me an article in German about Messner the climber.

10 July   Maria had quite a good swim, while I stayed within rescue reach. When she comes out of the sea, she often beams with delight and is most congenial. She tends to stop total strangers and tell them about the sea and its condition, and she nearly always lets them know that she is over 80. They smile and look interested, if slightly surprised, and make appropriate murmurs of incredulity and admiration at her age.

14 July   There has been another Maria 'disaster'. She says that 100 German marks that her sister had sent her, are missing and that I took them the other day when there was the fuss over the unlocked door. Logical argument and protestation are useless. She just says I'm ill and a liar. She also referred again to other items I've 'stolen'. The whole thing is becoming impossible. I really wonder sometimes if there is some sort of evil spirit at work mischievously mislaying things. Or does she sometimes imagine she's had things which she hasn't? Is it her way of making it easier for her to accept help from me? I wonder if when she dies she'll know the truth.

23 July   Life is becoming a perpetual exercise in endurance and patience, and the retention of a measure of cheerfulness. Maria is a constant problem and depressant, and it is continually sad to see. I can only hope that what I try to do for her does make things less bad for her than they otherwise might be – it doesn't seem to improve them. I do find it hard at times, but her total lot, I am sure, is worse than mine; as, undoubtedly, is the lot of many others, and failure doesn't mean I should not soldier on. If only I had some human help, or could talk about it to someone.

Later, when the Alzheimer's was fully developed, I realized that there were, of course, people with whom one could talk, finding through them some encouragement, advice and sympathy.

28 July Maria was very short with me when I raised a point about the home-help that she has occasionally. Soon afterwards, however, she thumped and apologized for being so abrupt, but she had, she said, such pain. Poor Maria.

After supper I watched a film with her. She was not any better. She said so sadly that she'd been looking forward to the summer, hoping it would help her to build herself up, but she can't walk properly, is mostly tired and in pain, and finds it difficult to think. Her sadness and disappointment are so deep and acute; and her depression is at times almost solid like a brick wall. I want to weep with the pity of it. And she has fought so hard.

29 July Maria thumped to show me with delight a picture of Princess Diana and baby in the newspaper. Despite everything, she still manages genuine enthusiasm over certain simple things that are good.

4 August Pondering on Maria's long struggle and present situation I thought how shockingly meaningless life can seem. All to what end? I feel that it can't be other than for our individual development linked to some later after-death purpose, plus being part of the evolutionary divinization of the world, as Chardin calls it. But whatever it is, it can be a very depressing, painful and frustrating slog.

12 August Normal life is not easy at the moment, not that it ever is particularly 'normal' now. As with the world, the abnormal tends to a greater or less extent to be the normal. Or rather, problems are routine.

18 August After lunch I had coffee with Maria and watched her playing Patience, which she has just learned. It's good if she develops this, though she was very slow at it ... I went to see Dr Sanders [her GP] about X-rays of Maria's left knee. He said they showed that there was practically no cartilage left and she had arthritis there. Maria was pleased to know what it was.

28 August   It was a lovely morning so I suggested to Maria that she might like to go somewhere and we decided to visit Dartmoor. It was a great success, even though her bad knee prevented her from walking more than a few yards. Her spirits on all such liberated and with-nature occasions are excellent.

30 August   I tried to discuss with Maria sending a package to Germany, but I couldn't make any progress. Getting her to deal with simple matters is like trying to get blood out of a stone ... I kept her company in the afternoon and we watched the birds eating.

31 August   Maria thumped. She'd lost a painting book and suggested that I'd taken it. I looked and found it in her bedroom. Why doesn't she look properly before bewailing?

2 September   It's a pity how Maria is, on the whole, dwindling. So does everybody, but it remains – at any rate pro tem – a pity. Although presumably pro tem doesn't mean a thing in eternity, it does mean something when you're in it and it is your only apprehensible time experience.

6 September   Maria thumped to cancel an appointment with Dr Brown. She has so much pain that she couldn't talk to any doctor. Mine's not to reason why, mine's but to do and cancel.

7 September   Maria wants to try to find somewhere by the front where she can paint waves during the winter. It is nice that she is so optimistic and positive. And today she seemed to be walking better and to be less gloomy. It often seems to be like this after she's decided to cancel something.

C.D. made an interesting remark about dealing with people who have depression. He said that the best one can do is to share it, so that the person can unload it and work through it. I've tended to feel that this is the case with Maria, hard though it can be. The sort of jollying along, 'buck up' attitude is, in his opinion, of no particular help.

10 September   As it was a perfect day, I suggested to Maria that we go to Golden Cap for a bit of a walk. She had had a similar idea, so we got Mrs Mason to take us there at 12.30, and, blow me down, we trekked until 5.30! The weather was beautiful and it was a lovely walk, but Maria, who was indomitable, only just made it. Her knee had seemed all right at first, but in the later stages it seemed two or three times as if she wouldn't be able to go on. However, going very slowly and with many rests, she made it back home and retired to bed.

She really enjoyed it not only for its own sake, but also for walking again over a well-loved and familiar area; and its morale-boosting effect was considerable.

The days now began to settle into a general pattern, of good fluctuating with bad, sense with confusion and, increasingly, German instead of English. I was gradually drawn deeper into my caring role and worried a great deal about Maria's plight.

24 September   Maria seemed reasonably spry and I took her to the bank. I then did some shopping, and when I got back she greeted me in a rather breathless state. She had slipped on the steps and, stumbling, had crashed against the glass of the door. Luckily, the glass didn't break and she didn't fall down, but I think that there may be some sprains and bruises. She wasn't gloomy about it and was grateful that it wasn't worse ...

I was about to read when Maria thumped to say that she'd fallen on the floor and was very dizzy. I helped her get a whisky and while she sipped it we talked and looked at the wind gusting in the trees. She then wanted to go to the front to look at the high seas. It was not too cold and seemed to do her good psychologically and physically ...

Maria thumped, wanting to show me something on television. This led to one of her moody sessions, when she can't be bothered about anything, but does not want to be alone; she just sits at the table talking to no particular purpose and, in such a mood, entirely unconcerned with what I might want to do.

1 October Maria was unhappy about the standard of chocolate, which she says is deteriorating. She doesn't miss much that is unsatisfactory [She was also ready to praise what was satisfactory.] After lunch I spent one and a half hours with her, just being with her in her valley of depression.

7 October Maria implied that I'd heard from Frances, who's been away, but that I hadn't told her. Dr Brown has told me that Maria had said that she'd been suspicious of everyone since her experiences in Germany during the war, and that she assumed that there was 'something hidden' in the most innocent happenings. She doesn't voice her suspicions in a hysterical way, but generally in a rather dignified, superior way.

8 October Went up to Maria patiently to play Patience – patiently, because she talks all the time in German, cheats mildly, is very slow and delays her moves.

9 October We had a good trip to Bridport. Maria bought a pattern and material for a nightdress, some toiletries, bulbs, and nuts for the birds. It did her good. She seems to have good days building up after bad days.

12 October I had coffee with Maria, who was cutting out the pattern although her pain did not make brain-work easy. I vaguely helped her.

15 October Maria was in good form and I was glad to hear that Frances had telephoned her. Later, Frances paid her a visit, which seems to have been successful, though Maria was not feeling too bright . . . As I was about to have supper, she thumped. She was in a rambling and forgetful mood, and I found it difficult not to become irritable.

16 October   We played a game of Patience, followed by an unusually interesting talk about mind over matter; and she explained the inspiration behind the best of her paintings. Despite pain, she was reasonably cheerful, but I wasn't pleased to hear her say that next week, if the weather is still like it is today, she wouldn't keep an appointment with Dr Brown.

18 October   Maria, seeming very low and dizzy, said she couldn't see the TV repairman arranged for this afternoon. Then – she changes all the time – she decided to go for a walk. Helping her is in a modified way what it must be like to be a secretary to a prima donna. We shopped and then continued down a lane and up a hilly field, which was an unexpected triumph for her. However, she still didn't want to see the TV man. She wants to do her hair and toe nails!

The TV man rang my bell to say that he couldn't get into Maria's flat. I asked him in for a cup of tea and a diplomatic explanation. In the middle of it Maria thumped and said that someone had been at her door. She then disappeared and didn't answer when I shouted through her letter box! I saw her briefly later on. She is in a poor state; she couldn't bend to cut her toe nails and she has a bad headache. I'm really at a loss in trying to help her and I feel so sorry for her; though I can't really condone her behaviour over the TV man.

19 October   I didn't have a good night. It is difficult not to be worried about Maria, not only her present, but her future. Then there are all the possible consequences of her condition and situation for me. Admittedly, we don't know the divine plan, but it seems such a gargantuan waste of our potentials in not being able to do more than just not be overcome.

20 October   As I feared, Maria isn't going to keep her appointment with Dr Brown: 'I can't go, I can't stand, I've been crying all night.' It's so sad. I did nothing but sympathize; anything else would be useless. I phoned Dr Brown, and he was as understanding as ever. I must just soldier on, trying to nurse her through the winter and indeed the rest of her life.

22 October   We went by bus to Axminster. It was a successful little trip, which Maria seemed to enjoy. She then gave me tea and started to talk about her sister and brother. Though I go on about her a lot, she really is an admirable person and, for the most part, surprisingly cheerful and lacking in bitterness considering all she's been through.

2 November   After lunch Maria felt like a walk, so we went down to the front and a little way along the beach . . . About 7.30 Maria thumped and said that there was a full moon, so what about a walk! So down to the front again, and very pleasant it was too, and not cold.

5 November   Maria managed to do some dressmaking. Later, I helped her finish a game of Patience, which she was playing to keep her mind off the pain in her back. She complained that Earl Grey tea no longer tastes properly. She so readily finds something to complain about when she has pain; it is, I'm sure, a partial form of defence.

10 November   I couldn't sleep well. I was puzzling about what line to take if Maria wants to cancel Dr Brown today; and then what the future holds for her, and so for me. I got up about 2.45am and made tea . . . Maria thumped at 5.15 to say that her bell had been rung twice at 4.45. She thought it was me coming to see how she was, but I assured her that it wasn't. She was thoroughly distraught; she must be near a breakdown, and there's nothing to be done about it. She says: 'At my age I can't face this sort of thing.' Why, in God's name – and I mean God's name – does all this happen? It's awful. I feel quite ragged myself. The devil is certainly at work. But why? And what to do? . . .

I phoned to cancel Dr Brown and the taxi. Then she thumped to say that she felt that she could go to the doctor after all. So I phoned to cancel the cancellations!

15 November   Maria came down and sensibly suggested moving a cupboard of mine in conjunction with other adjustments.

Maria still had flashes of excellent common sense despite her mental failures, which was sometimes very confusing for me.

27 November   I couldn't get any proper conversation out of Maria. This is not wilful; it's just that she is incapable of normal discussion at times. I have constantly to keep asking her the same thing or to keep it pending until there is a favourable moment; and it is often necessary to confine myself to a single matter at a time.

29 November   Her inability to communicate clearly, or at all quickly, in English is now becoming very marked and makes for ever increasing difficulties.

30 November   An engineer came to put in an extension to Maria's phone. I took him upstairs. Maria was slow in her movements because of pain; and I learned later that she'd got down on the floor in the bedroom to clean under a side table, and because of her knee hadn't been able to get up again. She'd had to go along on her bottom to the sitting-room, where she managed to lever herself up with a chair. What an awful business old age can be.

2 December   I helped Maria with her design for a bird-feeding house. She then had to retire to bed. Later I played Patience with her. It remains somewhat comic. She cheats fluently and half the time mutters away in German. But it's good that she has it as something of a mind occupying outlet.
  Shortly after supper Maria thumped to say that she had awful stomach pain and that she couldn't take all her pills. She was more or less crying. It was a small relief for her to have me up there to moan to. I do not use those words slightingly, for she's a tragic

complicated mess, with no apparent hope of ever being anything
else. Meantime, I am stuck with it, making endless efforts to help
her, but they are all more or less to no practical purpose; being
there for her to moan to is sometimes all I can do. What *is* the
divine meaning of it all? . . .

I'm delaying going to bed, and, indeed, I worry about going to
bed or to sleep at all. Not that I could do anything much for her.
Possibly I wouldn't even be able to get into her flat if she couldn't
manage to open the door. She ought to be in a Home, or have a
housekeeper-nurse. But where's the money for either, except
perhaps for a totally unsuitable former? Maybe I'll learn tomorrow that she's had a good night. Sometimes things appear awful
and turn out to be not so bad. But one can't bank on it.

In mid-December I went to stay with a friend. Going for a walk
one morning, I'd slipped on a patch of ice and badly bruised my
back, neck and ribs, so that movement was difficult and painful.
My host drove me home the next day. Maria rallied round and
insisted in helping me to take off my pullover, and gave me one of
her cardigans to wear instead, as it was easier to manage with my
bruised ribs.

During the following days, in which the pain and the difficulty of
moving became more marked and I had to sleep in a chair, Maria
continued to provide splendid sympathetic attention: she offered me
early morning tea, did some shopping for me, provided me with a
particularly soft eiderdown, massaged my neck, came from time to
time to see if she could help in any way and so on. She did all this
despite her own pains and troubles. I gradually became mobile again,
though not in all areas at once.

23 December   I sympathize very much with Maria's pain for
I'm finding mine difficult to cope with.

24 December   After lunch, I sat a while with Maria. She was
very low, with pain in her knee and a headache. I sat with her

again later, her headache being temporarily a bit better after some rum. But, as it seemed to be coming back, she decided to go to bed.

At this time I started to read a book that a Benedictine monk I knew had lent me. Called *He Leadeth Me*, it is a true story written by an American Jesuit who was imprisoned or in labour camps in Russia for fifteen or more years. It is a most sobering record and had a bearing on my Maria situation. Although it didn't help me practically at first, in due course its example of coping came to help me considerably. Not much later I also took encouragement from an extract from a book by the actress Joan Collins, which described how she coped with the brain damage her daughter suffered after an accident. She showed remarkable courage, effort and determination in helping her daughter to recover against the odds, and I found her positive spirit exemplary.

26 December   After lunch, I read more of the inspiring Jesuit's book. What a fearsome time he had. Compared with that, my recent pain and my worry about Maria, or certainly the former, are nothing at all. But it doesn't explain *her* suffering, physical, mental and, indeed, spiritual.

Whatever may be the way in which God's will may be involved for her, I'm sure that it *is* his will that I help her as much as possible. But that 'possible' seems to be very limited in any effective way. I can pray for her physical relief and, perhaps even more, for her courage to cope despite my doubts (perhaps lack of faith?) about the value of my prayers. I can also pray for my own guidance, wisdom and endurance. On the practical level, I can be at her beck and call, and do such chores as may help her. I can be with her in her valley of depression. I can help her with doctors and medication, though this is not always easy because of her inability to follow things through. But that seems to be really all that I can do. I can't engender any miraculous cure or relief.

30 December   Went to Bridport and collected some painkillers the doctor had prescribed and one or two other things for Maria. I have to keep doing what I can to add some measure of cheer and relief to her life, scanty though it may be.

1 January 1983   Maria is in a very low state. She hasn't been out since before Christmas ... She looks a very old sick woman – slow, hair untidy, and perplexed – the merest shadow of herself. Today does not auger well for 1983.

6 January   After lunch Maria thumped to say that she couldn't wash her hair because she couldn't bend her head. I felt a bit worn out myself, so I didn't stay long. Later I found her still in a poor way, but trying to be hopeful, though, apparently, she had almost been considering suicide.

10 January   Though she was tired, Maria was more alive, and has at last managed to wash her hair! ... She remained 'on the job' in the afternoon, but she had one of her 'troublesome' moods. She accused me of seeing Frances and not telling her (wrong) and of muddling up her prescriptions (the muddle was her own, while saying that *I* was stupid); and she upbraided me for not turning on the hall light despite the fact that it was broad daylight.

14 January   Maria wants to get a rectal douche to make sure that she's clean before and after taking suppositories. It took a long time for her to explain even approximately what she wanted – she knew no appropriate English words and it is an activity that is unfamiliar to me. However, with the aid of a dictionary and her vague illustration with the aid of a hot-water bottle and reference to a garden hose, I gleaned a rough idea.

We will go to Bridport for one tomorrow. I found it difficult to be patient with her confusion, impatience, forgetfulness and incomprehensibility, but I did my best. So did she, I reckon, for she made me an omelette and bacon.

15 January   I got up at 7.00am to learn that Maria can't go to Bridport, so I'll have to go alone. Anyway, it will save the cost of a taxi.

18 January   I'm beginning to feel that it is not right for me to
go out except for shopping and such like; and that I can do things
down here in my flat only when it seems all right for me not to be
upstairs. Not that it is her doing; it's just that I know that it's a help
for her to have me on tap.

23 January   Mr Green [a carpenter] called to plan with Maria
the making of the new bird-feeding house she has designed.

The bird-feeding house was an imaginative and practical invention,
and I still use it today. The best of Maria lives on in this and other
ways.

27 January   Frances came to tea with Maria. It went well,
though Maria had to lie on the couch. She talked a lot, but her
lack of finesse, her difficulty in making things plain, and in
listening to and understanding what is said can lead to confusion
and perplexity.

30 January   Maria thumped after breakfast and threw down
part of the morning paper, on which she had written, 'Don't
come to the door. It snow! – tiny!' And it was indeed snowing
very slightly. I tried to see if I could do anything for her, but she
was able only to put out the rest of the paper and to tell me not to
come up as she was 'very ill' and couldn't talk.

31 January   Considering the present difficult time, I found
help in thinking about the Jesuit in the Russian labour camps. It
became a point of honour with many of his fellow sufferers just to
survive each day. I must similarly aim to meet each day as a unit to
be survived. Of course, what I have to survive is far less hard and
painful, but it is often a struggle and a seemingly hopeless one.

1 February   I tried to explain Maria's telephone bill to her, but
she became exasperated at not being able to understand it; and
suspicious. She's apt to become suspicious about anything that she
can't understand, thinking that she is being cheated.

2 February   I spent most of the morning helping Maria to shift furniture and re-hang pictures. Despite pain, she managed reasonably well after a good dollop of rum . . . After lunch I helped shift more things until she couldn't carry on. We'll continue tomorrow.

3 February   There was much troublesome activity moving Maria's bed to another position and doing things connected with her electrical appliances. It nearly drove me mad, for I thought that so much of it was unnecessary. I was reasonably helpful, though at times I felt mildly explosive. But worse was to follow.

Maria accused me of having taken a coat of hers to give to someone. She says she never got it back when I'd taken it to the cleaners for her (if I ever did, for I don't remember doing so). She then returned to the old story of my having pinched other things. She says it's an illness with me. Actually, of course, it's she who is mentally sick, for her imaginings are quite wrong. It hurts me, but I *was* wrong in interrupting her accusations, in becoming irritated and in talking angrily. I ought to be totally dignified and quiet, though I do wish I could convince her of how wrong she is. Alas, there's no hope of that, seeing what she and her mind now are.

4 February   I had a poor night. I am so upset and despondent at Maria's accusations; at the deteriorating mental state that they reflect; at her pain; at her financial position; at her more or less absolute dependence on me; at her muddled flat; at the hopelessness of her future; at her growing handicaps; at the essential unhappiness of her situation; at all that I have to do and that I will continue to have to do with the many uncertainties that are involved; at the appalling sadness of her unrewarded courage and efforts, and at the way she has to undergo, so unjustly, all she has to undergo with no sign of release. Every day we both get older and our resilience is taxed more and more. And always nagging in the background is the disappointment that my continual prayers and the constant efforts of both of us don't work a miracle for her.

Well, I must grit my teeth and keep 'never doubting clouds will break'.

5 February   Shortly after lunch Mr Green came with the new bird-feeding house. It was an instant success. It fitted outside the kitchen window, and Maria was delighted with it. It is an admirable effort on his part, as was her original conception.

I was unhappy at being obliged to go away at this time, and considered cancelling my trip. But I thought Maria would not like that, and would feel responsible for stopping me. So I wrote two pages of instructions for her, and Frances and Edith kept an eye on her while I was away. I left on 8 February and returned on 23 February.

24 February   I went up to have coffee with Maria and Frances. I was pleased that all was OK and that they'd been out together. Other good news was that Mr Green had fixed a useful shelf in Maria's bedroom, and that the blue tits are using the new bird-feeding house in splendid style.

25 February   I talked with Maria for a while. She's as difficult as ever to talk to, as she rambles on in a not very clear way and keeps changing the subject. She really has deteriorated since a year ago.

27 February   I had troubled thoughts during the night; but I must keep hoping, and have faith in a loving God who refreshes us, and not succumb to gloom, hopelessness and self-pity ... Maria was quite bright on the whole, but very tired at times. She seems of late to be more tired more often.

She talked about visiting Germany, perhaps trying to end her days there in a Catholic Home. This would be a sound move considering her growing inability to communicate in English. But would she be acceptable now that she is British? And then there's the money question.

1 March   We went out, but Maria's knee was too painful for much walking. I hope something can be done about it; it will be a severe handicap if she can't walk much again, for she has been such a keen walker.

3 March   Maria rang my bell at 6.30am to ask if I'd rung hers around 3 o'clock when she'd been wakened by a sharp ring.

This odd electrical mischievousness, or hallucination of Maria's, continued to crop up from time to time. It can never have been an intruder, because the outside door to our joint entrance hall was usually bolted.

5 March   Maria had a very bad night, with pain in her knee and leg. She has pain whether she walks, lies or sits. She's tired and depressed at the hopelessness of everything. I can't see things getting better, and I feel far from happy about my prayers for her. They seem to be almost a waste of time. But I mustn't say that. How do I know what effect they may or may not be having? Pointless though they may seem to be, I must carry on with them.

6 March   Maria thumped as I was starting breakfast to say that she was going for a walk, which she did for twenty minutes or so. She enjoyed it and said that her knee was not too bad. Also, she'd had quite a good night. She is bewilderingly variable, for she's just thumped again to say that after the walk her knee is hurting again. 'But I wanted to find out', she added.

7 March   Maria took out some washing to hang up, which is a good sign. Then, after she'd made a soup for me, we went to the front and sat in the warm sunshine looking at the gentle sea for some forty minutes. She managed the walk, though with some pain, and she was cheerful.

The Second Period

3. 11 March to 24 April 1983

An incident on 11 March was to prove significant, for, in retrospect, it clearly marked the onset of the next, moderate, stage of Maria's Alzheimer's. I can see the evidence (amongst other things) in her subsequent increasing worries about security and her use of German, although as the extracts show, I did not for some time fully realize that she was actually losing her knowledge of English.

11 March 1983   We went for a walk along the beach and all was going well. It was pleasant and Maria's knee was not playing up. Then shortly before we were leaving, she tripped over a stone and fell flat on her face, without cushioning her fall with her hands. She cried out in shock. I couldn't help her up but was able to signal to two fairly hefty ladies, who came and supported her as she got herself up; and she was able to walk home slowly. The pain was mainly in her chest.

I tried to persuade her to call the doctor, but she wouldn't. Apart from supper, I stayed with her till 9.00. The pain in her chest, stomach and both sides was bad. I hope there's nothing broken and no damage to any internal organs. It is very, very worrying.

That this should happen when it was the best 'expedition' for a long time and when she fights so hard! I cannot pretend to begin to understand it from the viewpoint of justice or divine concern.

12 March   I felt I had to stay with Maria, as she was very tired and in great pain. It is very difficult to help her when she's so tired. She can't think or talk properly, and mostly she talks in German

... She insists on keeping her door locked so that I can go in and out to help her only if she gets up to open the door, which is the worst thing for her.

For the next three days Maria remained in a general state of pain, shock and distress.

16 March The phone went at 3.15am. Maria: 'I am very ill. The door's open.' I went up. The door wasn't open and she fumbled for a long time before she managed to open it. I don't know what had happened, but she'd moved things around and her clothes were in a mess. However, she can't explain anything and keeps talking in German. She got back into bed without arranging the pillows, so she had great difficulty in sitting up. However, after they were properly rearranged, she got on fairly well...

She surfaced at 8.30 and was in an awkward mood. She tottered into the kitchen. I tried yet again to persuade her to call the doctor, but all she could do was complain at being bothered when she was so tired. There seemed to be nothing to do but to leave her to it. She put on all the chains and bolts again, so there will be the arduous business of having to unlock. What the hell does one do?...

After a morning sleep she seemed marginally better. She's been cheered by a letter, which she insisted on reading to me in German. She still keeps jabbering in German, thinking, it seems, that I understand.

17 March Maria is unsteady on her feet, but by and large there may be a bit of an improvement, provided she'll be sensible (and I do wish she'd not talk so much in German) ... I was about to go shopping when she thumped. She feels bad again and now insists she wants to see Dr Brown. I phoned him and got Mrs Brown. She says he is very busy and I'll have to phone this evening ... Sat upstairs with Maria. She's very trying, fractious and changeable, and vague at times, but I'm really sorry for her.

Eventually, she prepared to go to bed, but I don't like her

locking the door with so many bolts, and having all the windows closed. I would have to get the fire brigade to break in if she couldn't open up.

I told her about phoning Dr Brown but I never know exactly what she's understood or what is in her mind. It's a sort of guessing game – but no game. However she sounded a bit brighter, and was speaking English.

I got Dr Brown at 8.30 and he'll see her next week. I went up to tell her, but she was in a terrible state, with new pain in her side. Eventually, I got her settled, and I'm now in her sitting-room, where I shall spend the night. I shall certainly get Dr Sanders to see her tomorrow. And it's all because of a stone on the beach! Maybe after this she will trust me more. Maybe the pain she's having now will, when it's over, make her other pains seem less. Maybe. Maybe. But it's no maybe that the battering she's had this last few months must have weakened her whole system, her mental state and her general powers of resistance . . .

Her sleep lasted only until just after 11.00. Then it was an awful time till 1.30am. She was unbelievably restless, speaking only German and continually rearranging her pillows. There seemed to be no logic in her efforts and I hadn't a clue as to what she wanted. Eventually she moved to the sitting-room and insisted on me leaving because she couldn't stand someone else in the room where she's sleeping. So I came down here, reluctantly, for she's so dopey that I feel she's liable to fall . . . I'm in a tunnel all right.

18 March   Couldn't really go to sleep in case I was needed. Got up at 5.20 feeling exhausted. Tried to perk myself up having a good shave. Refilled the bird bath; watered the plants, etc. just to do something while waiting apprehensively to go over the top of another day. Revised a note for Dr Sanders, whom I had phoned, asking his advice in case he can't get to see her – e.g., the door won't be opened; she won't be prepared to see him; she won't wake up . . . Sometime or other she thumped and I went up. She'd slept all right and was fair. Then unexpectedly a Dr Kilner, a locum for Dr Sanders, arrived. He examined Maria thoroughly. Nothing broken; it was a question of letting it heal itself; likely to take three to four weeks. He gave her some strongish painkillers.

I stayed with Maria for five hours, mostly watching television and listening to her German. She was moving more easily. I wish she'd remember to speak English. I hope she has a good night . . .

What a hope! I got to bed at 9.45, but was woken by a thump at 11.00, for no reason that I could discover; and it was a minor repetition of last night. Maria was tired, fractious and stupid, and speaking German all the time. She is really like a drunken idiot and so restless. So I came down at 12.15 for, probably, another ruined night . . . With her obstinacy, if it is that, at not speaking English, real communication is practically non-existent. And she acts as if I was at fault. It's a brick wall . . .

Shortly before 1.00am I went upstairs to hear if Maria was OK. I heard moaning noises and a cry of my name. I looked through the letterbox and shouted, but got no response. I then saw that a plant had fallen over and, though I couldn't see her properly, she was clearly on the floor. Exactly what I had feared had happened, and I had to call the police and, reluctantly, tell Mr and Mrs Woodhouse [the wardens]; reluctantly, because it's going to lead, I expect, to a revival of complaints about Maria's locks, bolts and chains; and perhaps even to her being regarded as not sufficiently able to look after herself to stay here.

A policeman came and, using a ladder, climbed up and broke in through the kitchen window. He found Maria on the floor. She was apparently OK and able to talk. With some difficulty he took her chain with the key on it from round her neck and opened the door. Then, after deciding nothing was broken, he and the warden got her on to her bed. The police cleared up the broken glass, and the Woodhouses talked about getting an ambulance and the doctor, but she'd have neither. They also implied that it was ridiculous to have a warden's services if the warden couldn't get in in an emergency. I can't quarrel with that.

I sat with her for a while and she was as awkward as before. I wanted to stay there all the time in case she wandered about and fell again. I also suggested she leave the door open if I came downstairs, but she wouldn't agree to either, so I had to leave her moaning and groaning at the pain.

She needs to be in some place till this is over. As for the future, I just don't know. From her point of view every day must be awful and she cried quite a bit when the Woodhouses had gone, though she remains very brave in her way. But oh dear!

There is no doubt in my mind, as I look back, that this fall, with its attendant trauma, coming after the one a week earlier, further accentuated the increased Alzheimer's that the latter had started. This is so, even though there were some better periods during the coming months.

19 March   I start today (now 4.25am) very tired: no sleep for two nights and an exhausting time. Sat around and vaguely dozed. Then, as a gesture against fate, dressed smartly. Thought of the possibility of putting her into one of the local Homes . . . I find this uncertain waiting about, and dread of her condition and attitude, and the whole awfulness of the situation, as bad as what hell could be.

After much debating, phoned Dr Brown and got him to agree that Maria should go into Winterbourne, his private hospital/ nursing home. He can see her there this evening. Phoned the hospital. They can take her, so I provisionally booked a bed. It's going to be damned expensive, but it can be worth it for both of us. Have now got to decide when to stir her (it's now 9.20), if she doesn't surface first.

She surfaced at 10.00. As I feared, she won't go. She's frightened I'll break into her flat. She more or less accused me of being responsible for her fall and definitely of having pulled the chain and the key off her neck and nearly strangling her. She must hate me for all the wrong reasons; it's awful for her and awful for me too.

Dr Kilner came – she spoke to him in as fluent English as I'd heard her speak for some time! – but he couldn't persuade her to go to the hospital. However, after various refusals, she suddenly thumped to say she'd go.

With monumental patience and trying not to put a foot wrong, I helped her pack and dress. It was terribly slow and changeable, but she was ready after four hours, which must have exhausted her as it did me. I had to phone the hospital three times to change the time of arrival. We got there around 7.00. It certainly is a well appointed place, and Maria was pleased with it. I didn't stay too long as she was desperately tired and the nurses wanted to do things. It looks promising, and the need for her to be somewhere under care is essential. I feel it may be worth every penny.

Maria remained in the hospital for six days. I stayed in a hotel nearby and visited her every day. She improved physically, but was still moody and confused, and in the end cried about not being able to go home. Dr Brown, who was worried about her mental condition, remarked 'She is not the lady I used to know'. However, he ultimately agreed, reluctantly, to let her return home, although he would have preferred her to stay a day or two longer.

26 March   Before leaving the hospital Maria ate a reasonably good lunch and was as pleasant as possible with the nurses, but when we were home it was hell. Mercifully, she hadn't lost her keys and we got into the flat all right, but from thereon she was muttering in German without stopping, rambling and repeating and repeating herself and being angry at her no English and my no German. I went downstairs for a while, but in no time she phoned and said (in perfectly good English) that her eye was hurting and what should she do?

I went up again. She seemed to have forgotten about the eye, but went on and on about something at the hospital that seems to have mortally offended her, quite wrongly I'm sure. Poor Maria! I just had to listen and be abused. However, she became quite solicitous when I pretended I'd damaged my back and she carefully applied liniment and bandage.

About now, I began, through local German-speaking people, to arrange phone calls and letters to Maria's relatives in Germany to apprise them of the situation and to see if a long-term solution could be worked out, perhaps in Germany; or if someone could come to England to help me sort things out. I was also able myself to communicate directly with a couple of the relatives who spoke some English. I stressed how traumatic the situation was, with its special complication of Maria's failing English. It was agreed that Maria's sons, Hans and Ludwig, and her sister Claudia would come over on 21 April to find out more about her actual situation (including financial) and to talk things over.

27 March   Slept very fitfully till after 7.00. Shortly after that, Maria surfaced and the rest of the day till now (5.30) was mostly an exhausting continuity of my coming down to try to do something, but almost immediately being summoned for various reasons. Because of the non-stop German it was exhausting – I expect non-stop English would have been almost as exhausting. The possibility of over-tiredness and another fall is worrying ... The whole business means that I can do nothing else at the moment except bits and pieces. And do I remain tired? I say a prayer from time to time, but being on the job the whole day is really praying ...

After supper I was about to go to bed when the damned woman (sorry!) thumped for absolutely no reason except to say there was a full moon, and then she chattered in German, without a single word of English, for forty-five minutes, tired and wandering around. She really is a lunatic on these occasions and unbelievably self-centred. But why, oh why, is there this German complexity? Please God! She needs someone to talk to and there is no one but me.

28 March   Oh! Telephone call at 4.00am. Will you come up? Not a word in English. All the lights on. Wandering about. Her heart was bad. Wouldn't take pills of any sort. Resented me pointing out what the time was – a great mistake on my part and thoroughly unkind. So she turned me out. I'm afraid she's losing her mind and nobody in this country could cope. And I, of course, am more or less mud in her eyes.

The day until now (2.45) has been real hell. She's been walking about and muttering the whole time, including an agonizing one and a half hours messing about with her bed and vacuuming the floor. She managed to make some soup, but her endless chattering, slowness and continually changing what she was doing was awful. She is now feverishly searching for her keys after suddenly deciding to go out. She locks up everything and continually mislays the keys ... She says she wants to go for a walk, but she won't make it, for I'm sure it'll take her an hour to find a coat.

She did make the walk, but German all the time ... On return she indicated she wouldn't thump again. But who knows? She thumped shortly afterwards to say that she'd lost some of her keys. I told her that she must have put them in her big brown handbag, because she had the keys when we came in. But then she couldn't find the bag. I told her she must have put it in the cupboard, but she pooh-poohed the idea ... In the end I left her to it and God knows if she'll ever get to sleep. I certainly won't go to bed. Talk about being driven round the bend. Poor Maria, I think she is. I really do.

29 March   Maria rang my bell at 2.30am. She was dressed and said she was going for a walk. I hastily put on shoes and coat (I had remained dressed) and caught up with her. We were out (full moon – any significance?) for over half an hour during which she stopped to admire the flowers in the moonlight. But she tottered and swayed and would, I think, have fallen three or four times had I not been there. When we returned, she said she was going to bed 'having been up since 6.00'. It was 3.10am!

30 March   A thump at 5.00am. Maria had a terrible pain in her side. I got her to take a painkiller. She doesn't seem able to take pills on her own initiative ... Had a protracted period – she side-tracked all the time – trying to explain about her money. She found it difficult to differentiate between her pension and her rent. She cried bitterly at one time at, I think, her sad plight and her loss of English, and she talked about her mother and grandmother. I found it difficult not to cry ... At times she laughs inordinately in a crazy sort of way. Is she perhaps manic depressive? ... I'm trying to learn never to raise a new subject in conjunction with an old one, and not to interrupt her, even if I can't understand.

31 March   A Mr Falk, who speaks German, came and talked with Maria for about two hours. He said she seemed confused and that she doesn't really know that she's speaking German ...

Went to bed early, but before long I heard noises and Maria appeared at her door ready for a walk. I had to put trousers over my pyjamas and totter up the street and back with her. She seemed to agree that I should spend the night upstairs and put blankets in the sitting-room for me and went to her bedroom. Hearing a thump, I went to see what had happened. The door was locked and she kept telling me to open it. She thought I'd locked her in, when quite obviously she'd locked herself in.

At last I got it through to her that *she* had the key and eventually she opened the door. She'd emptied most of her full wastepaper basket on to the floor. She then fiddled about with her front door and seemed to be saying in German that I had spare keys; and she insisted I go out. I refused at first, but I eventually went and have told her I won't come up if she thumps. I've just got to leave it be. Its very, very sad. What's more it's still only 11.15 – the whole night ahead.

The following two weeks were exhausting. Physically, Maria was reasonably well and was able to go for occasional short walks. However, she was restless beyond belief, seemed unable to concentrate, and was forgetful, confused and paranoid. She summoned me repeatedly, often in the early hours of the morning. At times she fought to remember her English, but generally spoke German. I got the names of a couple of German-speaking people, and arranged for them to visit Maria. I also began looking for possible Homes for her, preferably where someone spoke German.

13 April   The post brought a number of replies to my inquiries about possible Homes in this country. They were of no use ... When I was about to go upstairs to inquire about the forthcoming visit from Germany, I saw a police car arrive. It turned out that Maria had lost a 'locket' and she told the policeman that I'd taken it. She was quite confused and had to fight to speak to him in English. What hell it all must be for her. He came to question me, take my age and so on and asked if I was quite sure I hadn't taken it and didn't play games with her, like hiding her phone books as she'd also said. I gave him Dr Brown's phone number to phone him. Oh dear, oh dear, oh dear. I am so sorry for her; it's awful to see. She thanked him so politely when he left. After going up to see her again, he said that she'd now forgotten about the locket. I doubt if he's right...

She then thumped to tell me off and say, 'You'll see' and 'Our friendship is ended.' The lost 'locket' turned out to be the chain on which she hangs her keys and which for some reason she substituted with tape about three days ago. She said that I'd taken it when I'd 'half strangled' her the night the policeman had removed it after he had had to break in. When I said she had the chain on three days ago, she said, 'It's not true.'

14 April This awful business of her thinking I've taken the chain is as bad as ever this morning. She is convinced of it and is crying a lot. 'How could you?' she says. I cannot describe how distressing and impossible it all is; and how appallingly sad it is to see her so. It's hell for me, but I can accept it. But I can't understand why she has to be in such a plight. I can only hold on and pray for a miracle healing and that the chain turns up. Please God, reveal it and end this waste. Can you not please cast out this devil that's savaging her and her life and poisoning all her goodness? And it's such a lovely sunny day too.

15 April I had a bath at 8.30pm and in the middle of it saw that Maria had turned on the outside light. Then, lo and behold, at 9.00 it was the police again. Poor woman. Poor police. Poor me. This is getting really alarming. How can she be made to see sense? How can she be prevented from being put away? This time she told the police that I'd taken some money. They were quite nice about it. I told them to tell her that they were investigating and keeping an eye on me.

16 April   The police phoned. Maria had just phoned them again. The man couldn't quite understand and asked if he could have a word with the warden. I said better not as it would only disturb things. I'd have a word. I want to keep things going till Maria's relatives come.

After lunch, Maria came down and we had a brief conversation. Then – oh God! – the police car came again. It was once more about the chain; it really is a tragic mislay, for it was her mother's. The police just try to pacify her ... She rang the bell. 'Where is the yellow apron with my keys?' I went up and found it under some clothes. Then, 'Where is my bag?' It was sitting on the bed. Later, she thumped to say her television wasn't working; she'd just failed to turn it on properly. Then she suddenly said that I'd stolen £1,000 from her and turned me out with that maddish look in her eyes.

17 April   Maria said (in English!) that she'd give me time to repay the £1,000 at so much a month. Then suddenly it changed to £5,000 that I'd taken from her over the years. It's nightmarish. I have to cancel appointments for her with the chiropodist, the hairdresser and the bank. It is a perpetual muddle.

19 April   Maria thumped at 8.45pm and to my surprise had written a letter to Dr Brown in passable English asking advice about exercises to train her muscles – she's indomitable. Then, with my aid, she started rehanging some pictures, during which she suddenly blurted out again about the chain. I just remained quiet. She seems to be totally untired. However, at 10.50 I said it was time to go to bed and she let me out with an unsmiling face. No sooner was I in my bath than she thumped, but I didn't go up.

These awful bursts of feverish irrationality! They suddenly happen at an apparently reasonable moment.

20 April   I prepared things for tomorrow's journey to the airport to meet the relatives and for other things at this end. While I was doing this Maria thumped me seven times over a short period, once or twice for the same reason.

Maria's sons and her sister arrived on 21 April for a three-day visit. Maria unexpectedly decided to come to the airport with me in Mr Mason's taxi, which meant that, as the car could take only four passengers, I had to return by train. This was something of a setback to my plans as I'd intended to try to put them in the picture during the drive, including giving them some notes I'd had translated into German. I had had hopes of a solution in Germany, very much so because of the language problem. Maria too had for some time been wanting, and continued to want, to be settled there. But it soon became clear that her British naturalization would virtually make it financially out of the question. Basically, the object of the visit was to establish that in her changed condition she could remain as satisfactorily as possible in England, and that I was a suitable person to be responsible for her. They made it clear that if a private Home became necessary and Maria could be persuaded, they would consider contributing money as far as they were able, and that they would send me a next-of-kin's authority to manage her affairs. They went back to Germany on the morning of 24 April.

24 April   Maria was glum at first but became quite cheerful and balanced, except for speaking German, and said she must learn to speak English again. She is also anxious to hear from Dr Brown about the exercises to train her muscles.

4. *25 April to 23 October 1983*

The next few days continued in what was, sadly, normality for us. I looked through Maria's rubbish to see if the missing chain might be there, but had no luck. Dr Brown wrote to Maria about the exercises, but she tore up his letter and said she didn't want any at present. She kept getting muddled up about what day it was, what had happened, was happening and was going to happen. She'd ask questions that she'd already asked several times, including even her address, the names of her sons and her own surname. She also continued to lose things, particularly her keys, all of which, added to the strain of trying to communicate with her, was exhausting. Then there was another disaster.

30 April   Maria decided to go for a walk along the beach and, oh God, she fell again. This time, though, it was my fault, caused by my checking to see if her keys were in her coat pocket. I don't know how bad the fall was, but the atmosphere is awful...

There is a lesson for me here: not to be overscrupulously careful. Undue anxiety can do more harm than good and it can certainly set up psychological barriers of resentfulness and suspicion. It really was crass stupidity on my part.

As I look back, I can clearly see myself putting my hands in both pockets of her red coat while she continued walking, and her (reasonably) resenting it. In the confusion she stumbled and fell. It shows what a nervous state I must have been in. I did it because I was worried that she might have dropped the keys on the beach. It naturally strengthened her suspicions of me stealing from her. It was one of the stupidest and most unhelpful things that I did in all the years I looked after her. However, by some divine mercy, the devil was taking the day off, and there were no bad effects from that fall.

3 May   Maria went on and on, trying to work out her rent payments. [It was all quite straightforward and she had been doing it for years.] Things can be impossible on a practical level. The simplest matter can take hours to get clarified and even then she can forget it and it has to be repeated. She keeps on talking, hopping about from one thing to another; and she speaks loudly because she thinks that it's deafness that makes it hard for me to understand her German. Life is a vast slice of unproductive wasteland and, for her, it must be very frustrating and at times bewildering.

6 May   Maria thumped to go for a walk. It was a great effort on her part; but it was wearing for me, because she tended to stagger. I had to watch her feet and be on the alert to catch her elbow. On the way home she went into the church and we sat there for about fifteen minutes – a new development and a good omen?

11 May   Maria thumped me to ask the vicar's wife if she had any book that would help her to improve her English – actually she's spoken more English this morning and she really does try. She became demoniacally talkative.

12 May   We went shopping but she's getting so difficult to go out with, talking loudly and often in German, and being slow and confused. Yet she always smiles at everyone and says 'Hello' and 'Bye bye' with warmth.

16 May   Took some biscuits up to Maria, but she was searching for her keys. She's a perpetual minefield. She implied, as ever, that I'd taken them. What an exercise in compassionate patience, taking it on the chin and unyielding hope!

17 May   Maria talked non-stop in German for two hours, but she was on genial form. I managed to hold my own with the occasional word and appropriate expressions, though I understood very little. I feel that just to listen is definitely a help to her.

20 May   Couldn't sleep. I kept thinking that I might hear Maria thump, so I got up just before midnight. I feel that being up is some sort of gesture. It is kind of suffering on her behalf and hoping that in some mysterious way it will ease things for her...

Maria thumped before breakfast and was very poorly. She spoke near-perfect English: 'I want to go home and be near my boys and family.' It's so pathetic. And she's clearly very hurt by the way people say 'Speak English' and look at her as if she were a naughty child, and not an old lady who is just speaking her native language. She commended the vicar for the way he said: 'Excuse me, but I wonder if you'd mind translating.'...

Later, she was in her worst demoniac German-speaking mood. She talked (I finally managed to interpret) about writing to a store to get particulars of games that elderly people could play. This was to help Robert Coleman [an elderly neighbour], 'as he is so lonely'. She can have such nice thoughts and she tries so hard. This was followed by her wanting to teach me a game with matches, but she couldn't make anything clear. It was sad and frustrating. She also had lost her keys. When I found them, she implied it was because I had taken them. Oh dear, oh dear, oh dear...

At 9.05 she thumped and, blow me down, 'Where are my keys?'! The bloody woman – and it is what she is when the devil destroys her mind – had lost them again. We searched everywhere, except her handbag, where she said they couldn't be, so I just came down at 10.00, thoroughly frayed. It's quite hopeless...
She's just thumped to say she's found them, thank God, though

she wouldn't say where. It's a nightmare all right! When I was preparing to go to bed, she thumped again to give me some aspirin. She must have sensed I was in something of a state!

21 May   I broke down and cried at the whole hopeless situation: Maria's terribly sad dilemma; her, and my, unhappiness; and what seems to be the endless struggle for the future. I feel that she is like Lear with a similar loss of her native home and heritage, demented and wandering in a blasted heath with me as the fool, with the added dimension of no proper communication and her mistrust of me.

23 May   Maria said that she'd heard that Dr Brown didn't want her as a patient any more and that I'd said he was too busy to see her. There is no truth in either of the statements. She then talked about how unhappy she was. She's convinced I've stolen from her and that I'm a thief who ought to be treated for, as she says, 'such an illness'. She also says she's going to see the police to complain about how they broke into her flat...

She suddenly produced a rubbish bag full of discarded locks; there must have been at least a dozen. She was going to give them to the police, but she said that I 'mustn't be there' as she wanted to refer to my thieving and 'it might not be nice' for me. She'd already ordered the taxi, so we went in with Mrs Mason. I waited outside while they went into the police station. Maria managed to speak some English to the police, who took the locks, and some keys as well. They were somewhat surprised, particularly as she could have got some money for them, but she insisted and was relieved to get rid of them. Mrs Mason told me that at the police station Maria had referred to the thief as her nephew...

I phoned Dr Brown. Maria had phoned him and said again, half in English and half in German, that I stole from her, which he'd pooh-poohed. He said that there is no doubt that she's a bit paranoid. He was very sorry that he couldn't help her more.

24 May   I had a dream of standing in a road by a field sloping upwards with the sound of cars approaching and bright lights blinding me, so that I was crying out, 'Help me somebody, I can't see.' The dream certainly represents something of what I feel.

27 May At around 3.40am Maria put on her outside light and opened her door – I had been up since 2.45 – and was standing there with her phone book. Rationally and in quite good, though slow, English, she told me that she was wondering about phoning me, and then others if I didn't answer. She'd been woken with a clear cry from me of 'Come quickly, I'm going to die', and she didn't know what to do to help me. She was calm and totally rational, and obviously genuinely concerned.

I felt it was so strange that she'd had this experience after my dream the other night. We talked for about twenty minutes normally and congenially. She remembered certain appointments that were coming up and said, 'I thought I'd have to cancel them if you were dead.' After letting me out, she went to bed quite calmly. I found this curiously encouraging. It showed the goodness and concern of her nature and that, despite her own great troubles, there is a part of her that is still perfectly OK. Moreover, her talking and her looks were at their best. It felt *good*.

5 June I got up at 3.45am to read the Visitation of the Sick service, some marked bits of today's Psalms and a chapter of *He Leadeth Me*. Back to bed at 5.00. There is no doubt that saying these prayers gives me some measure of strength to keep hoping and trusting.

This spiritual boosting was virtually a daily routine. Prayers varied, but the Psalms were a never-failing source of help, while the Visitation of the Sick service in the Book of Common Prayer provided something that fitted Maria's (and my) situation; and *He Leadeth Me* encouraged me to fight and endure. Even though, for the most part, nothing may seem to happen as a result of prayer, one never knows what may be going on behind the scenes, nor what might have happened if the prayers had not been said.

7 June Looking at some X-rays, Dr Sanders said that Maria must have very bad pains (arthritis) in her back. I stayed with her till 9.45pm. She was in an extremely poor way, weak, in pain and depressed. The only sign of life has been a request for chocolate, which I went out to buy. She ate all of it and eventually tottered to bed. She seemed almost too tired to move. Also our relationship is in a bad state. She distrusts me, and my inability to understand her German irritates and depresses her. She must feel totally abandoned.

This distressful period continued for some days, though there were occasional brighter spots such as Maria playing Patience on her own initiative; defrosting my fridge for me; doing a few things in the garden, though wearing a fur coat over her nightdress and with her stockings hanging down, an untidiness that would have been unthinkable in the past.

11 June   At 10.45pm I noticed that Maria's front door was open and her light on. I went up to ask if she wanted anything. She was still fully dressed and said that her money had been stolen. She referred again to the lost chain and looked at me with cold eyes. What more can I do to prevent her going out of her mind?

12 June   It's incredible how she can change. Today has been as though last night had never been.

21 June   Maria thumped at breakfast time. She was in an awful state. Some brandy and rum that I'd bought for her had disappeared from their rightful spot. I think she was accusing me. I got a bit angry – after all I'd bought them – but presumably they are somewhere. [Although there are occasional references to various drinks, Maria was in no sense 'a drinker'.] At 10.30, as I was preparing for bed, she thumped and muttered something about me always being in her flat and about her lost chain. It is sometimes not easy to remain patiently compassionate.

22 June   I suddenly saw Maria going out. She didn't say a word. When she came back she asked me to phone the police (where she had apparently been) to tell them not to come as she was now not well. But at that moment a policeman arrived, so she said she'd see him. He hazarded a guess that she might be a bit senile. I'm afraid it is partly true.

24 June　I was alarmed when Maria insisted on climbing up a stepladder on to the garage roof in order to bind the rose bush branches. As well as climbing, this involved bending and stretching on a slippery surface. However, she managed it, though it gave pain to her back. There *seems* at the moment to be an improvement (though with lapses). She seems more like what she was before the fall.

26 June　Maria in excellent form; decided she'd like to go down to the beach and perhaps swim. We were there about two hours, then had some tea.

28 June　The devil has struck again. I went up to see if Maria wanted any shopping and she said the police were coming because I'd been in her flat while she was out, based, as far as I could make out, on seeing some of today's newspaper on her table. She said I'd left it there while she was out, whereas I'd given it to her before she went out. Then she continued, quite calmly, with the subject of my taking things from her flat and yet always pretending that I helped her, and referred to 'how we used to be friends'! She said the police wouldn't take much notice, because I was always nice to them.

I went shopping and the police car was there on my return. The policeman was about to drive off, but he got out and we talked. It's very saddening to hear him say 'She's crackers', and that they don't take much notice of her. And there's nothing I can do about it. It must be awful for her ... I did some gardening and Maria looked out of the window, instructed me as if nothing had happened and chatted in friendly fashion. Does she forget? It's very perplexing.

30 June　One miraculous blessing. Maria was wearing the long-lost chain. But she hasn't said a word about it or apologized, as is always the case when she finds something that I've supposedly taken.

6 July   After supper I tried to play a card game with Maria. It was a German game called *Skat*, but her rendering of it had nothing to do with the instructions in the book from the library. Nevertheless she enjoyed four games. I didn't correct her scheme of the game and, within the odd set up, she played more sensibly than I would have expected.

8 July   More and more when I see her good side, I am sure that she has been partially plagued by the devil, because her badnesses are so totally contradictory to her goodnesses; they often don't seem to come from the same person. My fight for her really is in part a fight against the evil of the devil.

9 July   After snipping things in the garden, Maria sat with me in the shade; and we played the new card game. She was in good form. It has been an encouraging day ... Later, she asked in her suspicious tone if I'd got her key. It shows one must never be over-optimistic or euphoric, just as one should never be the opposite.

11 July   Maria suddenly asked me for a comment on something in German. I had to ask if she could say it in English. But she wouldn't, and got into a real upset at my stupidity, and covered her ears with her hands in anguish and anger. So I just left. Five minutes later a thump; still furious and to say she did not want to be bothered with such a 'stupid baby'.

14 July   We played more of the ridiculous cards, still mostly without rule or reason. My interest remains to get her to win and to avoid her noticing my stupid play.

Another ploy I used was to try to get her out of the room, or looking elsewhere, while I arranged the cards before a deal, so that she got all the winning cards. I would then feign disgusted surprise at my rotten hand. Actually, the card games were for a short period a useful entertainment for her; and a reasonably pleasurable occupation for her was not always easy to find.

19 July   During my lunch Maria thumped five times (a) to say something about yesterday, (b) to tell me the wind was north-east, (c) to tell me her TV wasn't working, (d) to tell me it was and (e) I can't remember. But all in very congenial form . . . She appeared for an evening walk to the beach, from which we got back just before 9.00. There's no doubt she is better than she was, though not properly well. But this German is a profound nuisance.

20 July   We went by bus to Dorchester. She seems to manage trips again so that, apart from the German, one isn't very much aware of her being, or having been, ill.

23 July   We went to Bridport, though Maria had a headache. After a pleasant coffee, she was restless and incomprehensible in German. In the end, she was near to her diabolical worst and spoke most harshly, including: 'There's no point in your coming out with me.' So we meandered along in a sort of cold war state. Ultimately, she tried to be less 'inconsiderate' and I unearthed what she had been talking about and which I hadn't understood.

I could at times deduce certain things, or their general drift, but very much more, particularly detail, eluded me, and she could change subjects with bewildering and inconsequential rapidity.

29 July   A branch of the rose tree having come adrift from its moorings, Maria clipped it and tied it up. She did it so intelligently that you wouldn't think anything was amiss with her.

8 August   Maria had a spasm of fulminating against me because I had put out the rubbish for the Carstairs [neighbours], who are both not well. 'You like to be thought of as the nice Mr Hey-wood' or words to that effect; and then sarcastically she added, 'The *nice* Mr Heywood who steals my chain!' This was despite the fact that she was actually wearing it. The devil was in command for a few minutes, so I just shrugged my spiritual shoulders. Shortly afterwards, however, she was quite cordial. I've no doubt that I must be of some help to her even if only acting as a sink into which she can discharge her unhappy thoughts. She gets them out of her system to some extent.

10 August At times I view a hermit's life favourably, but that is not my assignment ... More and more Maria seems incapable of listening, of understanding or of remembering. She is, I fear, becoming increasingly difficult to cope with and to keep on an even keel; and she constantly demands attention. Yet she used to be totally capable of amusing herself and of generally coping on her own.

The days went on in this general fashion. Physically, although Maria's arthritis was always a problem, there were fine days when we went for reasonable walks on the beach and in the countryside, and made trips to nearby towns to shop or visit a museum. Communication continued to be a major problem. I am sure that when Maria was speaking German she often really thought she was speaking English. It was during this time that I began to take German lessons. Sometimes when I spoke to her in inferior German, she would answer me in perfect English. It was surrealistic.

To cope with Maria's constant demand for attention, I sometimes found it useful to ask her to show me how to do simple tasks (even if I knew how to do them), which she was usually able to do sensibly. But she continued to switch, sometimes at perplexingly short intervals, between being helpful and cordial, and railing at me for imagined injuries.

7 September Maria suddenly accused me of having stolen fifty Deutschmarks when she was asleep the other evening. These accusations not only temporarily knock the stuffing out of me, but the barrier they place between us is painful. They are also, of course, harmful to her; they detract from what I could do for her, and she is cutting herself off from what is virtually her sole human source of help. It must, too, poison her nature to some extent. I am sorely tempted to tell her to go to hell; but that would be against my duty. I must just take it on the chin and carry on trying to project a good spirit...

She's just telephoned to say that she wants to go to London tomorrow to buy a warm jacket. She spoke entirely in German, and when I asked her to speak in English, she said: 'But I am!' Her wish for such a trip is a good sign though.

We decided on the train for London and I arranged the taxi with Mr Mason. Maria then got upset about the trains, not believing what I told her, even when I showed her the timetable. Later, she decided that she wanted to go to Salisbury instead of London; so I had to rearrange the car and make inquiries about Salisbury and its shops.

8 September　The devil is afoot once more. Maria thumped to say that she now wasn't going to Salisbury. She referred again to me having taken her money and said it was therefore necessary for her to stay on her own.

I decided to go on my own by bus to Lyme. I phoned to tell Maria and asked her if she wanted anything. Yes – some coffee; and she thanked me nicely for phoning. Does she really forget what she has just been saying, for this sort of U-turn happens so often; or is she just trying to be forgiving?

9 September　I felt very restless and had depressing thoughts and sudden fear that Maria may really be going insane. I remind myself how often in the past she has had bad spells (often after goodish spells) and then come out of them. But she now seems worse than ever before.

13 September　After supper, Maria thumped to ask if I had any chocolate, so I took up what I keep for her. She didn't eat much and then gave the balance back with a cryptic remark (in German) that seemed to imply that I kept the chocolate to give to the '*kleine Fraulein*'. This was presumably L., who does some typing for me, and who is short, or, more likely, the newspaper girl. I have the chocolate in stock, of course, solely in case she wants it. Ah well! She can spoil worthy things. It's a shame.

14 September   Maria opened her door early and was in very congenial form. She wanted to show me some attractive old Christmas cards ... She paid me two further visits: to give me some drawing material, during which she had a go at an elephant that I'd done yesterday and which she turned into a slightly deformed specimen at the rear, and to give me a drawing book. Despite the opposite, she is so often generous and tries to be helpful.

Another knock on the door! She wanted to go for a walk, which we did. It was alarming at times. In her indomitable way, she insisted on going up slopes and along rough or muddy paths, and climbing through, under or over difficult fences and hedges. I had to watch her like a hawk at these obstructions and, indeed, during the whole walk. I kept ready to grab her should she trip over a stone or a rough piece of ground. And we had to battle at one stage with a strong wind. Going out with her can be quite a chore.

20 September   Maria, still seeming certain that she is going to Germany, wanted to know about the value of the Deutschmark and how easy it would be to transfer her pension ... She was in lively form and we played cards. I was brilliant, making sure that she won by playing with maximum stupidity and without her realizing the fact.

21 September   Mrs Harrison at the post office, who is very fond of Maria, says how sadly she has changed since she first knew her, when she was so full of life and vigour ...

Maria is in a generally weak and unhappy state today, though she tries not to give way. Despite what anyone may say against her for the past or the present, I cannot believe that she does not merit in her uniquely sad and difficult situation the maximum help that I can manage to give her.

24 September   Maria thumped as I was starting my breakfast. She was in her worst German-speaking mood. She was talking about E.L. and M.K. coming to tea this afternoon and for the *n*th time I had to tell her what their names were. She is making such a big thing about preparing for it, but I can't help admiring her persistence in trying to keep up standards of hospitality. When the ladies came, Maria talked in English all the time, though with some difficulty, and went out to their car to see them off.

25 September   Maria thumped to greet me with a smiling face and again spoke in English.

28 September   Maria called me on the phone at 6.15am to say that her front door bell had been rung twice. I assured her that the outside door was locked and that I'd been up for an hour and had heard nothing. It is odd how relatively often this has happened – four or five times in the last year. It must be some kind of dream or she's heard some other noise.

1 October   Maria, as far as I could make out, got on to the old chestnuts of me stealing money and having women in at night . . . I don't know whether to tell her to go to hell – perhaps, poor thing, she is sometimes there anyhow – or totally to renounce any defence against the injustice and hurt that I suffer in this hopeless morass. What would happen, I wonder, if I gave her up? I hate to think of her having to face her harassed life on her own.

3 October   After bringing me down yesterday's paper at 7.00am Maria tottered back upstairs, but though very slow, she was pleasant and smiling. It is this most splendid and admirable person – for at such times she really exudes real goodness – whom I cannot turn my back on, despite the devil that often seems to take over . . .

I went up to see how she was, which led to her talking with a surprisingly good memory about the Plantaganets and producing a book about them annotated in her thorough style. This minor resurrection was, I felt, quite something.

7 October   This German language business with her confused mind is so strange. For example, when I ask if *leben* means 'to live', she just repeats it. She then goes off into some sort of roundabout explanation (in German), not understanding that all I want is a simple yes or no. Then she says I'm an idiot. She doesn't seem to grasp that German isn't English, or that English isn't German when I speak it.

About this time I got in touch with Erika Hallward, a lady of German birth who was married to an Englishman and who, unknown to me, had met Maria before. Now, and for the rest of Maria's life, she was a great help, not only to Maria, in visiting and entertaining her, but also to me, in contacts with Germany and in explaining things to Maria in German.

11 October   A German-speaking English lady joined us for tea at Mrs Hallward's. They were both more or less spellbound while Maria talked away in great style.

16 October   I went up to help Maria prepare her rent payment. It was the usual up-against-a-brick-wall hassle. She is extraordinarily slow and blank about it, and she never grasps what's necessary nor listens to what you say. Earlier, I nearly exploded when she produced the receipt for her water charges and angrily accused me of having stolen it out of her bag. Ten minutes later she seemed to have forgotten all about it. However, such outbursts have been rarer of late.

21 October   At 6.40am I noticed that the outside hall light was on, so I went to see if Maria was in trouble. She'd just opened her door and she said that her bell had been rung three times at 5.00am and that she'd come down and rung my bell, had found the outside door open, and, when she got no reply to ringing my bell, had gone up again and phoned me, but with no reply. She wondered if I was ill or out. Very strange. I'd been up at 5.00 and heard neither door bell nor phone, and I hadn't unbolted the outside door till just before 5.30. There are various possible explanations, except for her bell being rung. I don't sleepwalk and even if the outside door had been unbolted, who would ring her bell at that hour?

Later, in the afternoon, she thumped to tell me off about not answering her rings this morning. She implied that I'd been out or had had somebody in. All afternoon she's been generally uncongenial. I'm afraid I became a bit annoyed, but she can be like a brick wall to talk to – no, more like a bulldozer coming at you.

22 October   Maria thumped twice around 5.00am. She was at her amiable best, smiling and calm, and showing me with great enthusiasm the full moon and the stars, which with the clouds were making a splendid sight. The light in her face on these occasions is really fundamentally divine – I remember a similar look many years ago when she was looking at a chestnut tree with 'its fingers' as she called them; and on other occasions. The good in her is so much more good than the bad is bad; and it is the real truth . . . When I was up with her during the afternoon, I nodded off in the warm sun. She suggested congenially that I'd been 'having an affair' the previous night!

23 October   Maria called me up to her flat to see the sun rising over the hill, truly a blaze of glory. I think I can honestly say that I've never before encountered such a totally perfect morning.

5.   24 October 1983
to 17 January 1985

For over a year our lives continued more or less as before. There were variations in detail but the overall pattern was consistent. Generally, it was a period of increasing deterioration and difficulty. However, it was not exclusively grim or gloomy; both Maria herself and events fluctuated, and the changes could be very sudden. Yet, though they virtually overlapped, the good and the bad were generally distinct.

In so far as it was possible, Maria fought hard against what was happening to her physically and mentally. She often showed real fortitude, and the goodness of her basic nature kept coming through. She would often be smilingly congenial and considerate. For example, she took flowers to a neighbour whose mother had died, and visited another neighbour who had damaged her leg and whom Maria, as a fellow leg-sufferer, sought to cheer up; she gave clothes to the lady who did some cleaning for me; loaned her precious Tudor scrapbook to others for their enjoyment; and gave a picture to Mr Coleman. She was concerned about Mr Carstairs in his ailing condition, despite an odd new obsession that I was going to marry his wife.

In stark contrast to her attacks on me, she was also periodically kind, particularly when I had a physical ailment. For example, she bandaged a cut finger till it was healed; she provided and applied a liniment to my sprained back; and did what she could to help me when I had an infected foot. This last problem, which largely confined me to a chair, coincided with a visit from my granddaughter and, in my limiting circumstances, Maria took considerable trouble to make the room ready for the occasion, including

putting flowers in it. She would also generally aim to draw my
attention to anything that was especially pleasing: a TV programme,
the moon and stars, the rising sun, the behaviour of birds. Never
during her illness did her spirit lose its deep admiration of, and
affinity with, the attractions of the natural world. She would try to
be, and, often was, methodical in practical matters, despite her
continuing confusions and forgetfulness; and more than once I
noted that she was smartly and tidily dressed.

None of these things, nor much of what follows, may sound very
striking, but they become so, and represent a fine spirit, when set in
the context of her continued distressing degeneration, disabilities,
pain and causes for depression.

Despite her disabilities, Maria would still walk to the sea front, and
occasionally go in the water; or she might manage a walk elsewhere,
perhaps combined with a trip in a car, or visit local places of interest.
She would go to tea or coffee with neighbours, or have them to her
flat. Because of her good-natured, outgoing approach, she would
generally manage these occasions, despite the language barrier.
From time to time she would continue to do gardening and a little
painting. The spirit behind her pictures gave them a special quality
that impressed me. She would still at times look at her splendid
history scrapbooks and, surprisingly, despite her general forgetfulness, she could remember certain marginally abstruse historical facts.
She also took pleasure in looking at her large atlas, which she had
heavily annotated over the years. She would look, too, at her
collection of books about the Himalayas, and at the booklets and
postcards about places she had visited.

We had a splendid trip to London on 23 November 1983. The
highlight was a visit to Westminster Abbey, a place of which Maria
was very fond and about which she had considerable knowledge.
While living in London and still speaking English, she had often
acted as a voluntary guide to other visitors. This last visit of hers was
strangely blessed. Not only was the Abbey uncrowded, but we had
the luck to get into conversation with a verger and then with
another visitor, both of whom spoke German. In the current circumstances this was indeed a bonus.

These positive moments were a welcome, if only occasional,

relief in a more generally negative period. Maria's arthritis gave her a lot of pain, and she was sick from time to time, 'spitting up food', as she said. These and her other disabilities inevitably tried and often depressed her, and she would cry and exclaim *'Ich kann nicht mehr'* (I can't go on any more). She once observed 'When you are 80 years old, you ought to be dead.' The cancellation of appointments was a constant fact of life, not because Maria was inconsiderate, but simply because she didn't feel physically up to keeping them. Pain and depression also played a part in an ever growing inability to amuse herself and in her need for company. They also, I think, helped to intensify her increasingly frequent confusion, forgetfulness and changeability. Repeated explanations could often fail to make her understand the difference between a bill and a receipt; she could no longer grasp elementary facts about her pension and rent; and taking medication was a hazard. She couldn't remember the names of people or simple objects, or places, nor her address; and at times she would switch from one subject, mood or point of view to another in a split second.

One example of her capacity to muddle things up was her persistent belief, based on nothing more than wishful thinking, that she was going to live in Germany, though the imagined ultimate how, when and where tended to vary. In April 1984 she was convinced that she was going to visit her sister and and brother near Munich, and see a doctor there, but when I checked with them on the telephone, they knew nothing about it. The flight she had arranged and paid for had to be cancelled, for the mooted visit never matured. It was a tragic incident, for she genuinely believed that the visit was a certainty, and she had hopes of its possible outcome.

Her security complex remained. She rigorously continued to use two locks, two bolts and a chain on her front door (which Mrs Mason likened to Fort Knox), and she had locks on her bedroom and sitting-room doors. She had all the locks changed from time to time. And as her confusion grew, she frequently found it difficult to open her door from the inside. It could be a matter of trial and error until she got all the devices released at the same time. The keys were frequently mislaid; and she would buy padlocks, though I never knew what she used them for.

If anything seemed to be lost (i.e., before she'd made any sort of search), Maria would accuse me of having taken it by breaking in or using a key that I'd copied. She also continued to accuse me of other things as before. This was, of course, very painful to me. Yet I could not but be conscious of her distress, because when she was in these moods, it was a real fact to her that I was a treacherous, lecherous crook with whom she was forced to consort. I did not really hold any of these injustices against her. 'This' Maria was ill and the 'other' Maria was good. I believed that as part of my task I had to accept the slings and arrows as an integral part of the 'good deed'! As I noted: 'It is not possible to *play* at being a sort of saint or whatever. The effort has to be wholehearted and unrelenting.'

Over this period Maria's slowness and her restlessness also increased. So did her frequent thumpings on the floor to summon me, often for very trivial reasons. Her speaking of German became more habitual, any English being only occasional; and, to a large extent, communication became 'a perpetual flounder', a sort of endless hit-or-miss twenty-questions exercise for me. It was, of course, as exasperating for her as it was for me, and because of my lack of understanding she would call me 'such a baby' or tetchily say, 'Why don't you use your deaf aid?' as if the trouble was that I was not hearing her properly.

The beginning of 1984 was marked by Maria's sudden belief that I had robbed her of £20,000, which, of course, she'd never had.

3 January 1984 Maria thumped after breakfast to throw the newspaper back at me and to snap at me for robbing her of so much money. This is going on now far, far too long. And it really is a form of madness. What can one do to prevent it getting worse? And if it does get worse, whatever happens to her? I feel almost broken by the constant injustice to me, the evil that she is suffering and the apparent hopelessness of the situation. I cannot possibly walk out on her, while I dread some stupid move on her part *vis-à-vis* the police or the bank. And all the time I can feel her gloom and misery, her isolated loneliness and sense of persecution and betrayal, both of which are so totally wrong. Then I remember the good Maria and it hurts even more that that good person should be tortured in this way...

On my return from shopping Maria appeared and said that she was going to the bank. She set off, walking slowly and grimly. It was a tragic sight. What can she usefully do at the bank? She returned after an hour, but made no contact with me. I wrote to the bank manager to explain her confused state and to ask them to be kind to her.

I wrote some notes for her, aiming to explain some points about the rent. At first she refused to take them and went on with 'Where is my money?' Later, she thumped and threw down some curtains that I'd lent her. This seems a really bad and, for her and her interests, potentially dangerous spell. Her mind is so obsessed, and if I write anything to her, her head is too bad for her to read it even if she accepts it. I just have to leave her *in extremis* and hope that she gets over it.

Things were slightly better when I took her up extracts from the paper and she spoke to me civilly; later she even said 'Thank you' when I asked if I could do anything for her. She said she was very tired and had much pain.

4 January   Maria thumped shortly after breakfast and we had a longish talk at her door. She was looking remarkably spry and didn't seem hostile, but I couldn't really understand her. It seemed to be about money, but I'd really no idea if it was still the missing £20,000 or whether I was to blame for something... She thumped again to ask me what day it was.

5 January   My God, I do need help. She's just asked me to give her back the money – the £20,000 – that I 'took off her table'. When I said that I'd never had such money nor had ever taken any, she said: 'You are a swine', and slammed the door. You can't reason with her. This is about the worst ever. Have faith!

It must be awful for her to feel that she has lost £20,000; to believe that it has been taken by the person she is most closely associated with and who is her only hope; to feel that she has no

recourse or source of help; not to be able to have proper communication; not to be well; and to have pain, and to see no hope
for the future. I pray that the hurt to me can count towards
rescuing her from the devilish clutches. What else can I do?

The police have just come. What *can* I do or say? ... They
stayed about fifteen minutes. She's bound to be disappointed that
her calling the police leads nowhere, as it must do; though it may
help her slightly to accuse me to them. But nothing can produce
the mythical £20,000 ... I cannot see friendly relations (such as
they were) being restored. The whole situation feels heavy with
doom. What a Merry Christmas and Happy New Year! But I
must not give way to self-pity or depression.

6 January   I put a note through Maria's door asking if she'd like
some of the food I'd been sent for Christmas. She came down and
refused, but did so in a very civil manner (and in English!). Apart
from the fact that she was feeling sick – and I hope she is also
spewing out some of the devil – she was as quiet and friendly as she
has been for a long while and it was a complete contrast to
yesterday. All this shows a positive refusal on her part to lie down
in the face of whatever it may be, and it was a great encouragement to me.

8 January   I wondered whether to go to church or not, because I don't feel like facing people, and it may make Maria think
I'm even more of a rotten hypocrite than she probably thinks I
am. However, I've decided to go. Not to go would be a minor
capitulation to the devil. I think the present traumatic experience
is deepening me to some extent. Perhaps that is part of its purpose.
I'm having to try to achieve a very difficult rescue of someone
who is in a very beleaguered and to some extent evil situation; and
I have no real cooperation or comradeship from the rescuee.
Practical steps to enable us to work together for her good, even in
the limited way that is at present possible, are restricted until she
stops believing that I've taken £20,000, and indeed stops thinking
she ever had it, two things quite beyond my control...

Delivered notes I'd made about the coming rent increase and

there now appeared to be no suggestion that I was too crooked to help her with such things, or that there was anything amiss with any £20,000. Later, with more like a resumption of diplomatic relations, she even let me watch her open her handbag.

9 January   A frosty morning, but at 8.30 I saw Maria go out fully dressed. There is no bus, so she must be going to a taxi that she wants to pick up without me knowing. It's pathetic to see her trudging off slowly with head bowed, perhaps embarking on some mission that may do her harm. I live on the edge of a volcano with eruptions major or minor liable to occur at any minute.

I heard her come back at 11.30. I went to ask Mrs Mason if she knew anything about it. Maria had been to a solicitor's. I said I thought that she must have had a long session, but it was not so long, because, having ordered the car for 9.30, Maria had turned up, as is her sad wont, at 8.30 and had to hang about for nearly an hour. Mrs Mason said there had been no communication between them, but Maria had spoken to herself in German now and again. I hope her visit was in connection with a will and not with something like issuing a summons against me. Oh dear! Sad day succeeds sad day . . .

Once again Maria wouldn't accept any of my Christmas food – 'Not till you've given me back my money'. This money is not like previous things that she's lost or I have 'stolen', but have then turned up, because this time there is nothing to turn up. That makes it more awful than ever . . . Suddenly she started up in German again. I couldn't really make it out except that she didn't like having someone like me living under her; I also got the impression that the solicitor would be writing about me to Erika Hallward, the warden and a relative of mine. What a jungle! Her manner was quite restrained. It was as if I was a naughty and rather despicable child who had to be reproved.

10 January   I took the morning paper up to her and I regard it as an encouraging sign that she hasn't thrown it back. What a reflection on the current situation. I also feel compelled, as just now, to hurry to the window whenever a car goes past to see if it's the police or Mrs Mason come to take Maria on some grim trip.

Maria thumped and said she had decided to go to Lyme by bus, but she wanted to sit by herself. When, after our return, I bought her some bread, she wouldn't let me into her flat but during the afternoon, she thumped twice and couldn't have been sweeter! And she gave me some stewed fruit that she'd prepared. These changes are very strange.

Then she thumped to ask if I had any chocolate. This is a bonus, because it represents a resumption of more cordial relations, which are so important for her.

1 March   After supper I had a pretty desperate two hours. Maria was in a quite unnecessary tizzy about something. Though I understood very little, she was clearly hostile. However, I managed to achieve what I hope was an anti-devil counter-attack. I stood there and said absolutely nothing, keeping up a barrage of positive remedial thought and feeling to the effect of: 'This is not the real Maria speaking. I don't accept what she says about me. God bless her. Give me wisdom to take the right attitude. Let me be a sink into which she can vomit all resentment, bitterness and disappointment.' I did that for over an hour and managed not to feel ill-will, hurt or self-pity. It was, however, a pretty savage hour, particularly as it was all in German. Perhaps, however, that was a good thing, as if I'd understood it all, I might have become more incensed or made some damaging rejoinders.

In the end she became much calmer and I ventured a remark in reply to one thing that I'd understood – I can't remember what it was. Thereafter we continued to talk amicably just as if there had never been this tornado and as if she didn't have anything against me. She even asked me to turn out the light so that we could look at the car headlights from her window. I feel that I achieved something of a victory and I'm sure that I helped her.

13 March   I went to bed at 9.00 and to sleep 9.45. But shortly afterwards, the telephone. Maria! I couldn't make out what she was talking about and she asked me to go up. She was sure that somebody – small children she imagined – had been walking up and down under the roof. Quite impossible, of course, but she was convinced though not frightened. I tried to free her of the notion, but no good.

The sadness of Maria's state affected me greatly. When the doctor said categorically that there was virtually no likelihood of her recovering mentally, I wanted to howl. In my mind I would question God's justice, and at times I wondered if I was justified in spending so much time and effort on such a lost cause. But the goodness that was still there, and her courageous efforts and other praiseworthy qualities never failed to convince me that I was doing right. Edith Bailey, referring to Maria's state, said: 'It is such a shame. She has so much to give.'

About this time I began to enlarge on the notes that I had made about her and what I did for her, so that they would be available if anything happened to me. I prepared notes in both English and German to explain certain things to her, and letters to be sent to Germany after they had been translated. The notes to her were really a waste of time. Even if I gave them to her or she actually read them, which was doubtful, they never seemed to produce any results.

The next few months remained a similar mixture of good and bad, varying in detail but not in principal or proportion. Maria's fighting spirit continued to show itself at times and she made some valiant efforts to maintain normal activities, doing her housework and some gardening. Once again she climbed up on to the garage roof to tie back the top branches of a rose tree. Considering her general condition, her age (82) and the height of the roof, this was really an astonishing feat, and she did the job very efficiently. During this period there were frequent visits by a visiting cat, or kitten as it was then. '*Die Katze*' would come running when Maria called from her window or would arrive uninvited; and though it was a cat of the largely impersonal variety, generally more interested, it seemed, in cream and/or a comfortable rest, than in personal friendliness, it gave Maria much pleasure.

Maria's incredible security complex remained unabated, as did her perpetual losses, which now included some new items, such as her clock, a pullover, her dentures, her purse, some spoons and a small bag. Inevitably, I was accused of having stolen the missing items, and, also inevitably, they turned up sooner or later. Strangely, these losses and accusations often happened after there had been in some other way quite a good day. Now and again she trotted out the 'old chestnut', harking back eighteen months to the way I had brought in three men to steal the chain from her neck. A new accusation was that I had tampered with her bank statement, because she didn't understand it and it didn't show the amount that she imagined should have been there.

At times, unhappily, we said some rather fierce things to each other. 'You who stole my money act as if you were king round here' was one of her remarks, and I, losing my cool, called her stupid. On another occasion when she was lashing out at me, I remonstrated by calling her wicked, to which she retorted that *I* was wicked. I should have known better, for, after all, I wasn't ill – she was; but there were times when it became too much for me and I lost control.

I was closeted with her for long spells, as she continued to need company. I felt, not surprisingly, that I was not a normal person living in a normal world. More than once I sobbed, partly at my own misery and partly at the tragedy of her condition. I noted too that I was becoming very thin. As to the outside world, I wrote that 'We may be becoming local freaks in the way we wander about and aren't really part of the local life with Maria speaking in German and me always in tow', and 'She's getting to be a sort of typical local simple old woman, particularly with her German. People look oddly at her or go out of their way to avoid her.' Sometimes, though, the people in the shops showed their own sadness when they remembered what she used to be and now saw the oddity of what she had become. Sometimes, too, I wished that they could see her at her worst and most difficult. I felt it would be comforting if others could realize the extent and nature of our particular hell when 'the devil had a field day'. But there were the other, better times as well, as when she was helpful to me when I had an infected foot.

11 July   I was about to get my breakfast when that woman! – dressed, with bag, coat and umbrella – rang the bell and said she was waiting for the taxi, as she was going to London. I pointed out that she was much too early – a trip to London had never been mentioned before – but she said that Mrs Mason was coming at 7.30 for the 8.04 train. I phoned Mrs Mason, who said she was coming at 8.15 for the 8.43 and that there wasn't an 8.04. So I persuaded Maria to come in and sit down, and I tried to ensure that she knew what to do about getting her ticket, her return train, taxis in London and so on. I also wrote down the train times for her and my phone number and name (not that she could manage to use a public phone). She didn't say why she was going. Then after a while, though she couldn't remember its name at first, she said she would go to Salisbury instead. Well, it's something that she's not going to London. [I couldn't go anywhere because of my infected foot.]

I arranged with Mrs Mason to make sure that Maria got the right ticket and to see her to the train. When she returned Mrs Mason phoned to say that Maria wanted to be met on the return train that left Salisbury at 2.35 instead of the one that left as 12.35 as she'd told me. I have no idea, of course, if Maria realized what she was arranging. I've asked Mrs Mason to meet the earlier train just in case. So I've done all I can. And now I hand over to God . . .

This sort of unpremeditated, unprepared trip is, to put it mildly, not satisfactory, especially with someone as confused and confusable, slow and vague as Maria, with her bad leg and probably no English. Let's hope that she gets off the train at Salisbury and remembers that it's Axminster she has to come back to. I meant to stay in pyjamas all day, but I am now putting on my trousers in case there's a crisis . . .

Mr Mason phoned from the station at 2.20 to say that Maria had not been on the earlier train. Ten minutes later a very nice man phoned from Honiton Station to say that he had a lady who was there by mistake. The lady was Mrs Maria Ritter. Clearly, she had been on the earlier train , but she had failed to get off at Axminster. The man said that he'd see that she got on the next train back and that someone would make sure that she got off at Axminster. The return train was, fortunately, quite soon. I phoned Mr Mason and asked him to meet it and please to go on the platform and make sure that Maria got off the train. What a good thing that I put my name and telephone number in her bag. Still, she did quite well in getting on to a train at Salisbury which was going in the right direction!

I have just phoned Honiton and thanked the man. He was very pleasant; he told the ticket inspector to see that Maria gets off at Axminster, and he's phoned Axminster. Very, very good service. He said she was a very nice person. And indeed she always is on such occasions . . .

When she got home, Maria said she couldn't remember the name of the station at first and then she couldn't open the train door in time. She came in for tea and we talked for nearly two hours. She'd bought a pair of comfortable shoes for her swellable feet, which seems to have been the object of the exercise. She'd also had 'something wonderful to eat with cream'; and she'd managed to walk from Salisbury station to the town – '*langsam*' (slowly) – and back. And she had enjoyed it all. But she is very tired. She said that she spoke German all the time. She agreed that it was a very good thing I'd put my name and phone number in her bag. And, oh yes, to crown her eventually successful trip, she found her key quite easily! I offer a small *Te Deum*.

Maria, in good spirits, thumped just before supper to ask me for some biscuits. It has been a successful day not only because of what she has achieved on her own, but because it has pleased her. Also – and this may be important – I never really worried about her. I had a feeling of trust and calmness.

Just before it began to turn dark Maria walked past my window. She was collecting a blossom from a tree. We chatted and she then went cheerily to bed. Later, she thumped to show me a fullish moon low over the sea, and then came down to tell me it was now behind a cloud. Despite all her rough edges, she has a genuine good childishness.

12 July Just before breakfast the unpredictable and currently intrepid Maria came to the door dressed in her wet weather hat and jacket to go and fetch the papers in the rain, both for us and for the Bullocks [neighbours] who are not well. Gallant and kind of her. She then went out shopping. She has certainly been un-usually active the last two or three days.

24 August Maria managed to do some painting. This was a good thing, though it made her very tired (and me too, actually, watching her), for not unlike her approach to life she often dashed at it without enough thought, and kept altering and functioning on intuition, which in life has not always been a good guide for her.

4 September Maria came down to say that one of her rings had been stolen and she asked me to go up, though I couldn't make out whether I was being accused or not. She then proceeded to produce some jewellery that I'd never seen before. There were two or three good-looking items. I was horrified at being shown them, fearing that they might get mislaid and that I would be accused. So, every time she went out of the room I went with her. Later, to my surprise, she gave me a costume-jewellery ring that had one stone missing. I didn't want to take it, but she insisted.

5 September Maria started talking about yesterday's ring. After a good deal of trial and error it transpired that she had given it to me to get the missing stone replaced, so that I could give it to Mrs Carstairs, as I'd said that I was going to marry her! I pointed out that Mr Carstairs was still around, but Maria said that she didn't think he'd live long and that when she'd asked me if I would marry Mrs Carstairs, I'd said yes. This is a supreme example of the awful language hazards. All I recollect is that once when she spoke about the Carstairs, she'd mentioned the word 'married' and I had thought that she was asking me if Mrs C. was married to Mr C. – I remember thinking that it was a surprising query – and I, of course, had said yes. Hence, apparently, her misunderstanding. This sort of thing is not only frustrating, but dangerous, and there must be many similar misunderstandings. To my relief, she took the ring back.

At this time Maria's son Ludwig and his wife, Helga, came to visit. Although, understandably, because of Maria's mental condition, there were occasional awkward moments, she enjoyed their presence; and they went together on a number of expeditions. It further pleased her when, on their return home, they phoned to say how much they had enjoyed their visit.

9 October Maria's painting today was an improvised doodle with constant alterations of colour and composition, all seemingly without any plan. She frequently put colours one on top of the other, in some cases I should think six layers (oil). There must be enough paint on that picture for at least four more. However, it was very good to see her working.

17 October During breakfast Maria either thumped or came down four times . . . She seems in a poorish way with leg, stomach and head. 'What can I do?' she says, poor lady.

In keeping with her hallucinations about people having affairs, such as – at various times – Dr Brown and Erika Hallward's daughter, me and Mrs Carstairs and others, she has just said that Mr Taylor [a neighbour] collects Frances in his car in the morning! Perhaps it's sometimes good that she speaks German and that no one understands her . . . Let's face it, we are still firmly in a darkish valley, in a tunnel, on the Egyptian side of the Red Sea.

15 November I'm writing this in Maria's bedroom at 6.30am, having been here since 9 o'clock last night. Just then, as I was about to take a bath, she telephoned to say she couldn't stand. I went up. The door was locked of course. But after I'd looked through the letterbox, she came into view slowly helping herself along on her bottom by pressing her hands on the floor. Mercifully, she hadn't bolted the door and managed to reach up and unlock it. She had apparently fallen and couldn't get up, and there was some nasty bruising on her right thigh.

Until 1.00am she tried, with my help and various chairs, to get up and into her bed. We tried in all sorts of ways and at various angles. I also tried to pull her along to the sitting-room, where the couch is not as high as her bed. But we couldn't achieve anything and she got more and more tired and miserable, and kept talking about the pain. Eventually, she went to sleep propped up on the floor, and I sat there in a chair.

This went on for half an hour, when she fell over on to the floor. Then, till 2.30 we made further fruitless efforts to get her into bed. All the time I kept suggesting that we should call the warden. She kept saying '*nein*'; and I was wary of doing so in case it might lead to an ambulance and hospital. By 2.30 I'd put some more cushions behind her and for the most part she slept, looking reasonably comfortable, till about 6.30. She did wake briefly now and again to talk about cold and pain.

At 6.30 she stirred properly and managed to sit up on the floor, but there was no prospect of achieving anything more. So I took the bull by the horns and called Mr Woodhouse. He came and, unaided, had her up and on her bed in one minute. Naturally, I'm exhausted. She was also sick in the middle of it all. Poor Maria. I do wish that I'd had the confidence to call Mr Woodhouse last night ... I spent virtually the whole day until 8.00pm upstairs.

This attitude of not wanting to bother people was always a fault of mine. I think that, as a general rule, one should never be slow to enlist available help when a situation warrants it, and shouldn't worry about inconveniencing others, especially as most people are ready to respond in an emergency. To allow one's timid or considerate reluctance to delay asking for help can be an unfair unkindness to a sufferer.

16 November   Maria seemed quite bright this morning and entertained the cat. She said her bruised leg was less painful ... Her lively condition is really quite remarkable at her age after the night before last, crawling about and exhausting herself for over four hours, and then sleeping on the floor. Her spirit seems remarkably cheerful at present ... During the morning, I took some shopping to her and was met with a totally inexplicable attack connected with 'the doctor' – inexplicable both in her German and as to what was amiss in her mind, and indeed what doctor. There is no doubt that she is not really sane. She has these

outbursts totally without rhyme or reason, or recognizable
relevance to anything. On this occasion it was such a sudden,
ludicrous attack that I walked out. I don't suppose I should have
done so, for I should remember that she is a sick person with many
troubles and I should let her vomit her spleen over me, being what
Dr Brown called 'the fall guy'. She soon improved, however,
coming down to bring me the paper and to draw attention to the
birds.

17 *November*   When I returned from shopping, Maria was a
flaming misery. I hate to be unfair, but being associated with her is
at times absolute hell. She moans and groans, is irritable, seems
dissatisfied with everything and I can't understand most of what
she says. Then she doesn't seem to consider me at all.

I wish I could submit the situation to some umpire and not be
left to fight on my own without any definite 'instructions'. I just
have to keep on hoping and to honour the principle of hope. But
however much I rationalize, think about my duty, trust, try to be
positive, etc., etc., etc., it is at times truly awful and I am most
unhappy.

29 *November*   I left Maria to go to the shops, but before I went
she came down and seemed to be complaining at my leaving her
. . . She really is going off her head, I'm afraid. Just now another
thump – she can't find the key of her bedroom door. Nor could I.
She more or less shouted all the time and wouldn't accept the
spare key that she had (surprisingly) given me yesterday, saying
that it was mine and nothing to do with her! She really is beyond
reason. She is becoming totally impossible about almost everything, except quite often, and rather surprisingly, when it comes
to doing practical things.

2 *December*   At 6.15am I heard Maria at her door. She was
trying to open it, but was getting confused with the locks.
Eventually, she succeeded and we had a mug of tea, in the middle
of which I went down to get some rum to put in it. When I
returned she was in the lavatory and there were some 'droppings'

on the hall floor. I was able to clear them up before she reappeared. She didn't seem to have been aware of them. [As far as I recollect, this was the first instance of the incontinence that was later to become prevalent.]

At 7.10 we decided to go to church for the 8 o'clock service, so I came down to dress. After forty minutes there was still no sign of Maria. Indeed, it wasn't till 8.25 that she finally came down. I knew that it would have been no use trying to hurry her or to suggest that we should not go. Walking was painful for her and, after the effort of dressing and walking, we didn't get to the church, as I'd realized would be the case, till they were finishing administering the Communion. This made her cry a little. However, people greeted her in a very friendly fashion and Mr Taylor offered to help to walk her home. The vicar also said, 'How nice of you to come.'

Of all the many sad moments associated with Maria, which even now make me feel like weeping, this was in its way one of the saddest. She had made a great effort to dress and to walk to church, she was aiming to do something good, and yet it all came virtually to nothing. It seemed like a very unfair divine rejection of her well-meaning, good and indeed brave intentions, and it must have hurt her.

While I was having my supper Maria thumped to say that she must give the vicar what she had been going to put in the collection in the morning. Then, while I was having a bath, the bell rang. It was Maria. I went out with just a towel round me (!) and explained the circumstances to her, now half way up the stairs. She laughed like anything at my appearance. Then, after my bath, she asked me to have breakfast up there. She thought it was morning! However, she became convinced that it wasn't when she saw the car headlights from her window. This made her laugh as well. In fact, she was cheerful and congenial.

4 December   *Du lieber Gott! Warum? Warum?* (Dear God! Why? Why?) I slept till 2.15am, when I heard some noise and went to investigate. Lights were on. I rang Maria's bell. She opened her door looking tired and dishevelled, and very slow. She had trousers and a greatcoat on. She didn't speak a word, not even when she'd made a mug of coffee, which she put beside her as she flopped down on the couch. I sat around and in due course put her mug into some hot water to keep it warm. Eventually, she launched into a tirade about having been alone ever since midday yesterday, which was quite untrue; and about me neglecting her, which was even more untrue if possible. There were also the other usual complaints against me. I made her some bread and honey and brought her the warmed coffee, which she consumed without a word of thanks, but just carried on with her tirade. She paid no attention when I tried to point out that she was wrong, nor did she seem to take in that it was 3.15 in the morning.

A little later, she put on a headscarf and started to go out, but after a few steps she turned back. She then more or less carried on as before until she said again that she'd go downstairs, or so I thought. But when I preceded her, she just shut the door. I phoned to tell her that I was staying up in case she wanted anything. I wanted to show her that she was not alone. She then kept turning the stair lights on and off. So here I am at 4.10 with coat, hat and shoes at the ready in case she goes out, hoping that I'll be given strength to carry on and praying for her as far as I can; and feeling far from lively or ecstatic! Is she disintegrating entirely?

Soon after, she did in fact come down and go out. I put on my coat over my dressing-gown and pyjamas and accompanied her. My presence was very necessary, for she was extremely tottery. Fortunately, it wasn't cold. She sat on a bench for a few minutes and then got up with my help. She then proceeded to walk on painfully, sometimes half stumbling. I think that, without me, she would have fallen more than once. I was afraid she was heading for the Taylors' house (4.45am!), so I was relieved when she branched off in the opposite direction. She never spoke except to mutter about her leg. I managed to persuade her to turn back. As we did so we met a cat (not 'ours'). This made a welcome diversion, for she called it to her, and there was mutual affection. She spoke rather loudly to it, but I don't think she disturbed the adjacent houses. We also had another minor bonus of hearing some waking birds beginning to chirp. When we got back, I asked her to come into my flat and I'd make her tea. She flopped down on a chair in my sitting-room and went straight to sleep. I carried on with some chores and said the Twenty-third Psalm to her recumbent figure. I hope it got through in some way. It's now 5.55 ... So begins another day.

Maria stirred shortly after this, had tea and some bread and marmalade. Then she suddenly produced a little bag out of her coat and extracted from it a silver cigarette case containing a lot of German marks and some English notes! She counted them out and I helped her to put them back. I gradually got her upstairs. Then just before I went for the paper, she asked me to go up again and she produced, wrapped up in a handkerchief, some silver spoons, which I'd never seen before. She did all this though she was very tired.

When I returned with the paper, she wanted me to go up for breakfast, and despite her tiredness she had already buttered bread for me and had tried to lay the table. She insisted in putting cream on my cereal. Then, quite exhausted, she dropped to sleep with her head on the table. Now, at 9.05, after moving there very slowly, she's lying on the couch.

I sat with her until she stirred at 10.30. I then went shopping. When I came back I saw Erika Hallward arriving; she'd said she might call. Erika stayed an hour and managed to talk to me before she left, having been given one of Maria's pictures that she'd said she liked. She said that Maria had not been very alert and had said that she was going to Germany, which Erika thinks is impossible. Maria was confused, said Erika, even when speaking German.

Meantime I'd started to clean Maria's frying-pan, which had got burnt. While I was doing this she came down to ask where her cigarette case with the money was. I said that she'd put it in her coat pocket when she was down here. '*Nein nein*', she snapped. So I went up and at once found it where I'd suggested. I spoke rather hastily to her (wrong of me, but it's so difficult to be patient at times). This made her cry, poor Maria. She's really like a baby now in many ways. However, I showed her how much of the frying-pan I'd managed to clean and we got on to finishing the job together in a reasonably happy way. I invited her to come down, to give her a change of scene, but after a while she went up again and seemed to want me up there. So here I am once more, while she sleeps wearing her heavy coat and feeling cold. I think I am almost totally cornered day and night...

I stayed upstairs till 6.30pm. It was all right on the whole until at the end she became irritated because I couldn't understand something she asked me in German. I must seem to her to be stupid and uncooperative. It would be nice, though, if sometimes she treated me with a bit more consideration, gratitude and warmth. I want so much to help her and am ready to do so, but I almost dread seeing her now because of her manner and her condition; and I never know what she is going to do next.

So it transpired. It's incredible. At 7.45pm, as I was getting ready for an early bath, down she came dressed to go out. I hastily put on shoes and coat, not having a clue whither away. It turned out that she wanted a breath of fresh air and for me to apologize to the Jenkins. [They were neighbours, and we had been due to go to tea, but it had had to be cancelled.] I felt awkward at bothering them, but they asked us in and we had a friendly chat for nearly one and a half hours. Maria was in quite lively form, though she had walked only with difficulty.

7 December   Just after 3.30am I heard Maria open her door. She appeared fully dressed. We had cocoa and tea respectively and talked for about half an hour ... Towards dawn, I heard her outside my door. I went to investigate; she was greeting the cat. I shut my door to prevent the cat coming into my flat, but Maria's right hand was by the door and her fingers got caught as I shut it. Why in God's name should these things happen to her? However, she took it in her stride – bravely I thought – and I went up for a cat-feeding session. But the fingers were hurting her. It made me feel quite sick, the way the devil does these hurtful things to her ... She has remained quite cheery and with no mention of her fingers.

I took to leaving my flat door open during the night, so that if Maria was in any trouble she could come and stir me; there was a joint outside door, which was kept bolted.

13 December   I was getting up at 4.20am when Maria appeared smiling and looking tidy. I sat with her upstairs for half an hour while she ate bread and marmalade. It was depressing. She was on about her stomach, her '*immer schmerzen*' (always pains) and how '*ischrecklich*' (terrible) it is. It's awful that all my effort and goodwill seem to produce no real amelioration.

She asked me why people were coming to tea tomorrow. The answer: 'Because you asked them.' Her reply: 'That's not true.' It's impossible with her today. Later, she rang my doorbell and walked upstairs immediately, reaching the top by the time I'd opened my door, saying as she shut hers, 'It's raining.'

14 December   Maria opened my door shortly after 4.30am. She said she'd had a coffee, and then went back . . . I must always try to impose on her such goodness as I can muster, be calmer about what tends to put me out. And fret less.

May and Donald Jenkins came to tea with her and the party went off well. Maria, speaking in German, was in sparkling form.

17 December   I dozed vaguely till 4.20am. Then I heard Maria stirring, so I got up and 'stood by' and wrote some Christmas cards. After breakfast she gave me a letter to post, and on my return I found her in a very cheery mood having had a beautifully made-up parcel from her niece Alexandra . . . Today has been on the whole a good day. She has been as congenial and cheerful as she was the opposite yesterday.

19 December   Maria appeared at 5.15am, cordial and bringing me a mug of strong tea. I'd already had two large mugs, so I've had enough tea so far to sink a small boat . . .

The day till now (4.20pm) has been very disorganized with a series of not unreasonable interruptions by Maria. She asked me again when I was going to marry Mrs Carstairs. Then an hour later she called me to go out and see if Mr Carstairs was all right, as she had seen him walking by laboriously! That action exemplifies her kindly thoughts for others, not to mention her confusion in implying earlier that Mrs Carstairs was available for wedlock.

20 December   I helped Maria to put up one of her Madonna and Child pictures outside her front door. It looks good.

21 December   Maria surfaced briefly off and on after 3.45am, including one short nocturnal walk to look at the stars. Unlike them, she was not very bright.

24 December   Maria thumped at 5.45am. She was dressed and controlled, and just wanted to talk. She wants to write to Hans's 'nice' wife, Magda, who is in hospital.

After lunch, she set out to post a letter to Magda, but the wind was so cold that she had to give up. I took it for her. I hope it reaches Magda, but it will take some time over the holiday period.

Christmas Day   Maria surfaced early, but did not seem at all bright, and said she wasn't going to church … Later, she came down dressed and seeming composed. Shortly afterwards she came down again to say she had a visitor, and there was the cat having bread and milk … In the end she went to church. Thereafter the day was rather confusing. We went to the Taylors for a morning drink. As it was raining, I thought we'd better take a taxi, even though it wasn't far. Waiting for it might make us a bit late, so I phoned Mr Taylor to tell him. Then Maria started to walk on her own despite the rain. She also apparently thought that we were going to the house next door to the Taylors'. I caught up with her just as she reached this wrong house, where there was no reply. She then tried to get to the Taylors' through some under-growth. However, I eventually steered her there, both by now slightly damp.

The Taylors had their family for Christmas, and their grandsons were opening presents. Everyone was friendly, and coffee was served. There wasn't much chance to chat, but Maria liked it. We left after forty minutes and the Taylors' daughter drove us home. Maria has been today, as on the whole in recent days, mostly balanced and congenial.

This was gratifying, because Christmas had always tended to be a rather sad period for Maria. She missed not only the family get-togethers that she had known in her childhood, and later before she came to England, but also the traditional German Christmas celebrations.

26 December   Slept very well till Maria came down and woke me at 3.15am to say she had some tea for me. She was full of goodwill. I went up and we chatted for about an hour...

I was getting ready to go to sleep when Maria appeared to tell me that she had some books for me. I went up and she presented me with twenty to thirty paperbacks. This is a typical example of (a) her kindly thoughts and (b) her lack of understanding in broaching it at that time of night.

28 December   Yet another early start, with Maria appearing at 4.00am. She believed that I or somebody else was in trouble, and she wanted to see if she could help. That was about as far as I could understand. '*Komisch*' (Odd), she said...

After lunch, Maria was indecisive. Her habit of just sitting and making no move to do anything, and my not being able to get any suggestions out of her or to understand what she says, can be trying. However, I came down and was about to write letters when she appeared quickly three times: kindly to see if I'd washed up; to ask me to come up and help find her glasses, which I found at once lying on her couch; and to weigh a letter to her brother, which I then took to the post office.

29 December   As I finished breakfast, Maria thumped and there she was, dressed and with her bag, saying she wanted to go to Dorchester, without thinking about when the buses went. However, I succeeded into talking her into postponing it till Monday. She then insisted on going to buy some flowers (me

paying!) for Mrs Taylor. On return, she produced a postcard to go
with the flowers and managed to write her name and a message on
it. And down we went. We were received cordially and given
coffee. Maria is at present in remarkable (and almost, at times,
exhausting) form.

31 December   I managed to make something hot for Maria's
lunch, but she kept talking incomprehensibly, though I think it
was about flying to Hamburg. She then talked about furniture
disposal. She suddenly seems to believe that she is going to leave.
She indicated that she needed cash to pay for the flight. But how
can she fly to Hamburg? Who'd meet her?

I'm worried about her current restlessness. She seems so excessively on the go. I'm particularly worried about this talk of going to
Hamburg. How is it going to be prevented, because I'm sure it's
not based on any arrangement at the other end?

New Year's Day 1985   After breakfast Maria interrupted me to
ask what a certain envelope 'meant'. On looking inside, I saw it
was a will. As soon as I told her, she snatched it away and
hot-footed it upstairs.

It's been a confusing day since then with Maria, still seemingly
thinking that she's going to Hamburg, talking about packing and
wondering what to do with things. I was mostly upstairs from
11.00 to 6.00 doing things for her. In the early afternoon she had
wanted me to get a taxi to go to the Hallwards, though I couldn't
make out if she was expected. I managed to divert her by ringing
up my number, but pretending that it was Mr Mason's and saying
there was no reply, and then going out ostensibly to another taxi
man and saying he wasn't in.

Mercifully, Erika Hallward phoned me to ask if Maria was in
fact going to Germany, as she had said she was going to Hamburg
on Thursday and so couldn't go to tea! It is all wishful thinking,
and sadly worrying. In the event, Erika asked us to tea tomorrow,
which suits.

2 January   Maria came down about two and a half hours before it was time to go, dressed and ready. I had to try to keep her 'amused', but I was disappointed to hear further talk of packing and travelling. Eventually, she became so restless that I rang up Mr Mason to ask him to bring the car early and take us for a small trip before we went to the Hallwards. Once we got there it was a great success. There were three members of the family there and another couple with two young girls. Erika was very nice to Maria, who thoroughly enjoyed the children and the family atmosphere, with the big Christmas tree. Erika had time to tell me that Maria had remarked, 'If it can't be arranged to go to Germany, then I can't go!' On returning home, Maria was full of how nice the visit had been. She was very cheerful and hinted that Germany was out till a more suitable time in the spring.

3 January   Maria thumped in something of a state of shock. She had had a notice of the death of Hans's wife, Magda, to whom she had written just before Christmas. Magda was 52, and had died on 21 December.

When I had mailed that letter to Magda, I had, oddly, wondered if it would ever reach her. Sadly, it never did, for she had died even before it was posted. Her death was particularly sad, for she and Maria had a real mutual affection, despite not having seen much of each other. Magda was also a good and kindly correspondent, sending friendly letters to Maria from time to time; and I remember how nice she had been when I telephoned her after Maria had fallen in March 1983, for she spoke some English. There was also that strange, though retrospective and perhaps muddled, occasion on 28 December when Maria believed that I or somebody else was in trouble.

4 January   Maria talked again about going to Germany. Nothing is arranged and I've no idea whether she has permanent residence in mind, or just a visit, supposing either is viable, which is doubtful. One mercy is that she doesn't plan to go till after Easter...

5 January   A cold morning with a white frost. At Maria's instigation I looked at a splendid sunrise; but this was immediately followed by her coming down and saying that I'd taken a ring out of her wardrobe. She soon appeared again dressed for the cold weather and wanting to buy some chocolate. I accompanied her. She was in good humour and made no further reference to the ring!

7 January   Maria came down at 3.00am and woke me to look at the high, full moon. This was followed by tea and a cordial conversation upstairs till 4.20, when she went to bed again. I went to bed again, but she interrupted me at 5.20 with the cat and the information that there was snow on the ground. Now, at 6.05, I'll get up for good! A positive start to the day though.

After breakfast and before I realized it, Maria was hammering away at the ice on the bird bath, to make sure they had something to drink. Thereafter until now (3.40pm) it's been mostly a typical Maria-oriented day.

8 January   Maria rang my bell at 6.10am, smartly dressed. I was due at the dentist at 9.30 and she seemed to think that she was going too. When I emphasized that it was only me, she seemed to sulk. It's impossible at times.

After getting the paper, I told her that I'd decided to cancel the dentist, but she was still aloof and gloomy. What does go on in her mind? It is all so dispiriting, these bouts of confusion; the apparent disappointment for, or my seeming rejection of, her; and her antipathy to me for no reason. It's such a shame when, despite her childlike enthusiasm, something seems unnecessarily to dampen everything for her. Her irritating restlessness continued and I found my patience sorely tried, coupled as it was with her incessant chatter and muttering to herself. She decided that some of the snow should be cleared up and she valiantly insisted on doing quite a lot of the shovelling herself! It was icy underneath, and I had to stand near her in case she slipped. She then more or less forced me to go upstairs. I think this was just to sit with her, but I never know what's really in her mind. She's now trying to thread a needle. I can't settle down to anything. I'm sure I'm to blame for my reaction, but I feel like crying 'How long, oh Lord, how long?'...

Maria came down to tell me that she had phoned Germany and, as far as I could make out, had asked someone to find a room for her in Germany. Subsequently she was in a totally restless and confused state. She kept turning the TV on and off and was confused as to what date, month and year it was. She was generally difficult and unpleasant, and clearly very unhappy.

I've no idea how to handle this situation, and because of the language problem, we can't even talk properly. I really don't know what to do about going to bed tonight... Well, I'm going now (9.20), having just woken up after flopping on the kitchen table.

10 January Woken up by Maria at 2.30am and went up for a coldish cup of tea and a talk till 3.30. I then managed to sleep off and on till 6.00, when she woke me again. I gave her some chocolate and we had a brief cat interlude down here till 7.00.

When I came back with the paper, she was dressed and *determined* to go to the dentist! It was, of course, far too early. She kept wandering about, so eventually I rang Mr Mason to take us... In the event, the trip was successful. Maria got it 'from the horse's mouth' that the dentist didn't want to see her again!

Later, she kept bumping, either restless or complaining. Though I criticize her, I acknowledge her many qualities and the difficulties that she has to cope with – ill health, old age, relative loneliness and gloomy future outlook. I also acknowledge my own impatience and self-concern on occasions, my sometimes ham-fisted handling of things with perhaps some cowardice, and my lack of cheerful trust in God. There is also my frequent negativity. Life is one long lesson, often learned slowly and painfully, and often perhaps not learned at all. But I wish some intelligent angel would give me a book of instructions on how to handle her!

Got to bed and asleep by 9.30. But – oh dear! – she came down and woke me at 10.15; and I went upstairs. In an effort to get her to take sleeping pills, I took half a one myself and said that I was tired. At this, she insisted on me sleeping on her sitting-room couch, providing me with two blankets. So I got comfortably to sleep by 11.15 hoping I was set for the night.

11 January   But no! I slept all right till just before 2.00, when Maria appeared fully dressed and seemed to expect me to get up, for she started to do things around the flat. So, very sleepy, I've come down.

Managed to sleep till 5.30 when Maria appeared at my bedroom door with the cat. Thereafter she kept coming down from time to time for no apparent reason except that she can't keep still. And when I go to the dentist again, she wants to go too. This means another taxi, for she can't go by bus. Talk about albatrosses ... When we returned from the dentist – she'd enjoyed the car ride – we sat and talked, now in a totally amiable way.

13 January   Slept fairly well till 4.15am, when Maria came down. I took my tea up, while she had coffee. She gave me some good buttered rolls and we chatted amiably till just before 6.00 ... From breakfast onwards until now (1.45pm) it's been pretty awful. She kept constantly coming down, to ask me what aspirin is; to ask me to write to the doctor, but no questioning could elicit which doctor or where; to talk about her sister Claudia now 'being in the area'; to say something about me being married; to raise the question of a furniture remover. Most of it was so unrealistic, not only on the basis of what she was talking about, but also in the details of that unrealism – the unrealistic within the unrealistic.

I was alarmed to see that she was taking down pictures in the sitting-room, apparently with a view to moving. Please God, don't let her go right out of her mind. Tried to carry on as calmly as possible. The opposite only does harm to her as well as to me.

17 January   Not a good night. I was up twice with a headache, then Maria stirred me at 4.45am to say it was '*Ganz weiss*' (Quite white): more snow. I went up with a cup of chocolate for her and we looked at the scene and talked till just before 6.00 ... After breakfast I brushed away the latest snow; Maria came down to lend me her overshoes. I had to crush my toes into them, but I did so because I wanted to make her feel helpful, for that was her intention ... On my return from shopping she said that she wanted to exercise her leg muscles and buy some chocolate. She achieved this quite gallantly, though I was continually anxious about her slipping and concentrated on being ready to catch her...

And that, if I'd realized it, was about the last of even marginal normality on her part; or of such marginally normal association between us. The definite last, severe stage of her Alzheimer's, though it lasted for over the next two and half years, was about to begin.

The Third Period

6. *18 January to 31 March 1985*

---

18 January   Maria woke me at 3.45am and I took hot chocolate up to her, but she was not very well. She really does need to be looked after ... As I finished breakfast, she came down and sat in the sitting-room and dozed a bit...

What a black day. Went to shop, not taking too long, except for a few extra minutes to have a radio fixed for Maria. When I got back, there she was, lying outside my kitchen window, half on the grass, half on the flowerbed, wearing only her night-clothes and a housecoat, with Miss Miller [a neighbour] bending over her. Miss M. said she had asked someone to call the warden. Maria, in her most impulsive but well-meaning way, had taken out her rubbish bag, and, in the icy conditions, had slipped. She seemed in pain in her stomach area.

After about ten minutes during which she was moaning, with an occasional apologetic brave smile, Mr Woodhouse came and did his valiant act of slowly, and with much pain for her, managing to walk her to my flat and to a chair that I'd put with high cushions by the sitting-room door. She sat there till Dr Sanders came. He thought she'd broken her femur. He rang the casualty department at Weymouth hospital and arranged for an ambulance.

Maria spent only one night in the hospital. Although the X-ray revealed that she had cracked her pelvis on both sides, she demanded that I take her home. She was so insistent and made such repeated efforts to get up and get dressed that I asked the doctor if she could be discharged. He agreed on condition that there was someone to look after her and someone who could lift her. So we returned home at 5pm on 19 January.

20 January   It wasn't too bad until 00.40 (!), when Maria woke up. I got some dozy sleep, but had to keep popping my head in and out of her room. From then till 4.00 it was another misery of poor Maria trying to get up; putting on shoes and jackets and taking them off again a number of times; fiddling with the bedside phone and reading off the numbers '*Ein, zwei, drei*', etc., and once trying to make a call to Germany, till I stressed it was the middle of the night. And always she was talking and crying out at being in an awkward position (not that I blame her). At one stage I got her a cup of tea, and I think one reason she wanted to get up was to go to the toilet. What the answer to that is I don't know. There's the difficulty of getting her both to stand and to walk.

She got tired by 4.00am and slept till 4.40. It was the same all over again till 7.25, with the slight variation that she didn't want me to stay by her all the time. But she kept on trying to stand up, showing in the circumstances great spirit but not much realistic sense. She dozed again, but I've not been able to persuade her to take any sleeping or painkilling pills. Her cracked part is, of course, very painful.

In retrospect, I wonder if it might not have been better to have left Maria in the hospital although she so clearly hated the idea of it. Probably I should have; but I can say that now because I know with hindsight that she was going to have to go there anyhow, and when it then happened it was an unavoidable 100 per cent certainty, whereas, at the time, there seemed to be a slight possibility of managing her at home.

I'm very tired (never took my clothes off all night) and once when I was mildly *non grata*, I stood outside her door for an hour just keeping an eye on her to see whether she'd manage to get up, so that I could dash to avoid her falling ... She dozed till 9.30am. I also asked the warden if he could come round and help her to the toilet. He came in five minutes, but, in the event, as moving is still painful for her, I brought a commode upstairs. It proved of use, though Maria had slightly wetted her bed in the night. We covered the bed with a towel and he helped her to get back on to it. He then persuaded her to take two painkillers...

After he'd left she kept wanting to go to the bathroom and did manage to stand up by herself; but I persuaded her to wash in the bedroom. I got water and soap, and various cloths, all after much guesswork. She then had a little to eat, and she's now (12.40pm) sleeping again. On the whole a promising morning. But she's mentally very vague...

Maria slept till 3.00, but we soon had the sad, tired end-of-the-day restlessness, with the changing and rechanging of everything. Had to call on Edith Bailey to help things along. Afterwards, I couldn't get Maria to bed or to take pills. Had to call Mr Woodhouse again. He achieved both, and she went to sleep about 8.15. I'm staying the night up here. Maria wants it. I don't suppose I'll sleep much. How can I? I hope she does. The thing that worries me most after her mental state is the fact that she can't go to the lavatory and is very unhappy about wetting herself and/or using the commode.

21 January   I slept fitfully – in clothes except for trousers – looking in at Maria three times, and seeing her legs gradually coming out on to the floor. At 2.15am the old no-go situation began. It is almost impossible, and I'm exhausted before the day starts. I had to get her in a sitting position on the edge of the bed and leave her with a bucket at her feet so that she could do business. But it was, of course, quite impossible and she refuses to use the commode.

The whole thing is quite hellish, both for her to suffer and for me to see. Over and over again she tries to get off the bed, then tries to lie down. She gets more and more tired. She asks for things, or for things to be done, which are wildly stupid or contradictory or repetitive – get the bucket, take it away, fill it, empty it, put it in the corner, bring it back ... It's now 5.15am and this particular hell has been going on for three hours. Maria can't even get into a comfortable position lying down. We try and try; and then up again. Of course, I'm useless at this sort of thing, but I can't keep calling on people at all hours of the day and night to help shift her a few inches...

It's now 7.30 and the only real let-up was when she sat quietly having one and half slices of bread and butter. There's just been another hassle with me trying to get her to use the commode; and with her trying to get up and walk to the bathroom. She managed to sit up about twice out of some thirty efforts; and she had to dry herself and her nightdress where, poor Maria, it was all wet. Our bodily evacuation system is staggeringly inefficient at times. One ought to be able to turn a tap on and off and that's that...

I don't think of the future any more. I just try to concentrate on each moment and keep going ... Now 9.30 and since breakfast things have been a little better. For instance, while I was out of the room, she took off her two wet nightdresses and put on two fresh ones. Then, after I'd made other excursions, I found she'd managed to stand up on her own. She did a few more stand-ups, but she couldn't walk. By this time she was very tired and ready to be in bed, where she was apparently comfortable. So I escaped to phone the doctor and ask for the district nurse.

During all this Maria kept ringing the bell [a small hand bell by her bed] for me, and wanted me to phone Ludwig and Helga in Germany. I did so, and she had a chat with Helga. She then got back into bed, and thoughtfully told me I ought to have a sleep too ... The warden's told me that he's asked the district nurse to bring incontinence pads...

Maria woke up at 11.45 and thereafter we had a hellish four and half hours, during which, because of continuing incontinence, she wanted to get to the bathroom, refusing to use the commode. She managed to get to the hall, but got stuck by the sitting-room door. She was unable to progress, though my help and that of chairs (which I put near her to grasp) were available. Over and over again she said she couldn't make it and sat down on one of the chairs; or she said she would go back to bed; or would go to the sitting-room instead. But over and over again she could manage only the same one and a half useless steps. I nearly screamed at her 'stupidity', though admiring her spirit. And three times she made messes. It was quite awful for her. And she kept muttering '*Kinder, Kinder. Nicht. Nein*' (Children, children. Not. No), presumably feeling the added pain of her sons not being with her...

She was still stuck there in the hall, when a lady from Social Services arrived. She tried to get Maria to go with her, but Maria was budgeless. Then the doctor arrived. Without much bedside manner, the two of them made a cat's cradle and carried Maria to her bed, despite her cries. This was a godsend. They both told Maria that she must stay in bed as that was the treatment, and I managed to get a few stronger painkillers from the doctor. They also both warned me not to ruin my health.

Everyone stresses that Maria is naughty not to do what the doctors say, and they are right; but she does it because of her spirit and because of the hell of incontinency.

After they'd gone, Maria became quieter and quite pleasant; and she took two of the new painkillers and two sleeping pills ... I must be unreservedly kind with her, no matter what. She is such an unhappy and forlorn person and deserves to be loved, blessed and praised.

The next eight days continued in much the same difficult, sad way, with Maria, constantly restless, getting up – and getting stranded – and lying down, moving things, putting on a multitude of clothes on top of each other and taking them off again with bewildering frequency, mislaying items and, of course, accusing me of taking them. She began to have stomach trouble and her incontinence was complicated by diarrhoea. I decided to switch her to Dr Kilner, who lives near Erika Hallward, and began to make tentative plans for her to go into Lyme Regis hospital.

29–30 January Maria had difficulty in moving during the night (28/29). More diarrhoea. It's hard to keep pace with clean clothes. Harder for her to stand up. I fear for the future. I can hardly talk on the phone for crying. Dr Kilner suggests that she might be terminal ... The 29/30 night is quite appalling. No sleep. Pain. Moaning. Couldn't or wouldn't take pills. Phone Dr Kilner at 3.30am about it. He suggests to crush them in honey. They stick in her mouth. We sit on edge of her bed for over three hours. I call the warden and he gets her back in; later, the district nurse fixes her up more comfortably. But only for a while.

These thirteen days that followed the fall on 18 January rank in my memory as perhaps the worst for both Maria and me during the whole period of her illness. What followed in the hospitals, where she was now obliged to go until she returned home, was also very severe (particularly at the beginning), but perhaps not quite as bewilderingly, despairingly, hopelessly and utterly exhaustingly traumatic as those thirteen days. They live in my memory as having a special concentrated hellish dimension.

31 January At 5 o'clock yesterday evening a whirlwind descended in the the form of Dr Sanders. He looked at Maria's stomach and decided immediately she had a swollen bladder and must go at once to Weymouth hospital for examination. This really put the cat amongst the pigeons, with everything arranged for the evening and for hoping to get to the hospital in nearby Lyme. I had to run around in circles collecting clothes for the night (for both of us), getting Edith Bailey to be with Maria, phoning the warden, working out what to do about keys and so on. And far too soon an ambulance arrived. We reached Weymouth between 6.30 and 7.00.

Maria had over a gruelling hour having her bladder emptied – at times four nurses on the job, I think. She yelled from time to time. It was awful to hear. When it was finished, the doctor told me that there would now be a period of getting her bladder to operate, and rehabilitation in walking. I told him about Lyme hospital and couldn't she go there? He said not now, and that as they hadn't a bed free, she'd have to go to Portland hospital. This was a blow. So to Portland by ambulance, with more lifting and shifting of Maria.

When we got there (blowing hard and pouring with rain), Maria was put in a single 'room', one of a number opening,

without doors, on to a central passage. My request to stay in the
room for the night had to await the senior night nurse. She was
very cordial and arranged for a kind of bed to be made for me
alongside Maria. Maria was given something to make her sleep
and we were both off before 10.00. I was at a loss as to what to do
about getting her to Lyme. (Portland had no objection to her
going there when a room was available.)

Slept quite well, and so would any sleep be by comparison with
recent nights. We were given tea early in the morning. Maria was
reasonably perky. Breakfast was served – excellent meal. Then
during the day I stayed around doing what I could to help the
nurses help Maria and to help her myself, pushing the Lyme
hospital option, and waiting for the doctor. He came around 1.00.
He explained that Maria could go to Lyme if a bed was available.
Otherwise, he said, she needed care and rest. Maria has been very
restless and cried a lot, but though she has pain in the pelvic area,
she shows signs of standing better.

The day staff were as splendid as the night, and the head nurse is
taking great trouble to try to cater for Maria's quite special needs. I
phoned the warden and Mrs Hallward to put them in the picture,
and stayed with Maria, for what it's been worth to her. She is in a
really unhappy state, not least with the lack of communication
and the pain. She's eaten and drunk somewhat better ... It looks
as if she'll have to stay here, and it may be better than another
change if she really settles in.

At about this time I became too preoccupied, distressed and exhausted to keep up my diary in full, and all I have is memory and
single-word reminders. These indicate that it was a very traumatic
period. I recollect that I stayed the night of 2 February at the house of
one of the night nurses, who kindly gave me free bed and breakfast.
Otherwise I stayed in one of the male wards, which had a number of
spare beds, spending all day with Maria.

She was for the most part very unhappy, and cried more than once
'*Wo bist du, Gott?*' (Where are you, God?), though the nurses
were doing their best. There was also some antagonism on the part
of other patients to Maria's endless chatter, for which I tried to

apologize. The hospital treated me very well in letting me stay with her, feeding me and giving me a bed.

There was a visit by a geriatric consultant, who spoke German and who told me that Maria definitely had dementia. He was the first and, I think, the only geriatric consultant who ever saw her; and this (apart from Dr Brown's earlier belief) was the first categorical diagnosis of dementia. I also recall Maria's (and my) introduction to the catheter for the passing of urine, to which she reacted very adversely; though they tried to dispense with it, it became permanently necessary.

Maria was transferred to Lyme hospital on 7 February, and during her first week there I recall mainly her perpetual restlessness, a great deal of correspondence; arranging visitors for her; and the beginning of several weeks' daily visits to the hospital from 2 to 8pm (the visiting hours), with the first of the subsequent daily bus journeys followed by a toilsome uphill walk and, soon, a routine whisky at a pub on the way and a prayer at a small chapel (double spiritual fortification), as I girded up my loins to face, always, I am ashamed to say, with apprehension, what might have to be met with during the next six hours.

I was able to resume my diary on 14 February. Maria remained confused, unintelligible (even in German) and distressed at being forced to stay in the hospital; she simply did not understand the situation. Although her walking was improving, she continued to have bladder trouble, was constipated, wouldn't eat much and drank less. Her reluctance to drink, which became habitual, might, I think, have stemmed from the trauma of having her bladder emptied. Consciously or subconsciously, she might have been avoiding the risk, as she saw it, of a possible repetition.

Edith, Frances, Mr and Mrs Jenkins and various other friends came to see Maria occasionally, and both the vicar and the local Catholic priest arranged for a number of German-speaking visitors. Erika Hallward; Grace Weston, a local schoolgirl; Gretel, a young German lady who lived near us; and Miss Marffy, a former nurse, all of whom spoke German, were frequent visitors. Maria was cheered up by these visits, but it was clear that her mind was wandering and, for the most part, she was unable to make intelligible conversation. She also began to do odd things, such as pour tea into the bowl holding her dentures, try to widen a hole in her shawl with the end of her spectacles, put her sandwich into the milk pudding and pour tea over it.

I kept Maria's flat clean and the plants watered in the hope that she would be able to return. At Dr Kilner's suggestion, I phoned Nurse Anna Gordon, who then worked at the hospital, about possible home-nursing. They both thought that Maria might eventually be able to manage at home if she had nursing help. Anna became a key figure both in organizing Maria's subsequent return home and in enabling that return to be maintained till the end of Maria's life. I can still remember her sympathetic attention to my call, and can hear her saying, when I told her of Maria's distressing times, 'Oh, the poor lady!' Also, I now embarked on what proved to be an endless series of grant-seeking letters to charities, anticipating the cost of nursing help when Maria returned home, although this did not come to pass for some time.

9 March   Stayed with Maria from 2.00 to 8.50, when they put her to bed. I must say she weathered sitting up all that time in a chair very well, and she was not *too* downcast. She managed to look at some books and magazines. She looked at one of the magazines about five times in succession without a break, just turning over the pages...

She smiles splendidly at all visitors and at the nurses, and as Frances, who looked in, says, she has a smile that includes her eyes even more than was the case with some of her past smiles. Perhaps something valuable is taking place within her.

In mid-March Dr Kilner indicated that Maria might be able to go home for a trial period on 1 April. She wouldn't need a nurse for the whole day, but he said there should be one on duty throughout the night. Maria's walking was not too bad; the problems with her bladder and her bowels were associated with old age, and she would probably have to have the catheter for ever. He confirmed that she had dementia and would not improve mentally. He also arranged for her to come home prior to 1 April for part of a day, accompanied by an occupational therapist.

18 March   Anna told me that she'd been given a week's leave of absence for when Maria comes home, and that Maria's day visit was planned for next Friday, for which she would need clothes. I'll have to get a lot done, so that there is nothing wrong and plenty right with her flat.

19 March   A disappointment at the hospital. Anna had been sent home with a bad back and they didn't know when she'd be able to return. I phoned her mother, who said that they wouldn't know for forty-eight hours whether it was 'only muscular' or something else; nor whether Anna would be able to come and nurse Maria on 1 April. This is worrying for, if Anna can't come, it throws all the plans out of joint. This illness of Maria has been an administrative minefield, apart from anything else...

I've been told that an ambulance will take Maria to the flat on Friday and that I'm to bring her clothes on Thursday. After the visit I should take the clothes back until her proper discharge. I was also warned by a kindly nurse about home-nursing. Apparently, it can be very uncertain. For one reason or another the nurses may not turn up or cease to be available – cars can break down; snow; they can become ill or pregnant; and so on. And there is no cover as in a hospital. The point was well illustrated by Anna's sudden back trouble.

20 March   Erika Hallward and her daughter came, and I got Erika to tell Maria in German what was going to happen on Friday. Erika said that Maria was much more lively than last time, but her German still made no sense. She was totally confused: she apparently didn't know where her home was and seemed to think that she didn't have one.

21 March   Took in a case with Maria's clothes for tomorrow. Maria seemed to understand about tomorrow, but she began to be crotchety and to fiddle with things, including her urine bag and attachment. This was briefly interrupted by a visit from Mr Hornby [our local vicar], who couldn't make head or tail of her, and whom she seemed to ignore at times. He said a prayer, and she managed an 'Amen', but when he'd gone, she said something, which seemed to be 'Why does he talk for God?' ...

After supper, she was worse except when I told her that Dr Kilner had confirmed the going-out arrangements. She lit up at this for a time. But she then kept asking me questions in German, which I didn't understand. This upset both of us and I became infuriated with her when she fiddled with, and pulled apart, a special shawl that I had lent her. Moreover, she said it was hers! Then, as so often, she accused me of this and that. One day I might suffer the last straw and bash her more than verbally, which I sometimes do in my mind. I'm also tempted at times to walk out on her; but that would be a dereliction of duty and I would very much regret it ...

Phoned Mrs Gordon. Anna expects to be working again on Monday. That is good news. But I can see that Maria may be difficult at home.

22 March   Maria arrived at the flat just before 11.00. She was accompanied by two physiotherapists, and the ambulance men carried her upstairs. The visit was definitely a success. Maria was bubbling over. She recognized the flat and knew her rooms. She was also able to walk around unaided. She insisted on me making coffee for everyone, and laughed and smiled all the time. Finally, to my surprise, she made no difficulty about going back to the hospital around 12.00. She had her urine bag on, but it was adjusted so as to make mobility possible. I reckon that if her ebullience is still there, Maria could be a handful when she gets back permanently; and may not be all that happy at having people around ...

I went to the hospital at 2.00. Maria seemed pleased about her visit and at the thought of going home for good, though I wonder if she really realizes the latter ...

Miss Marffy came at 5.30 for about half an hour. She found

Maria somewhat more coherent than at her last visit, and understood her to say that she does not like being asked a lot of questions, nor is she willing to do anything if a lot of people try to persuade her to do it. This could, perhaps, have something to do with her not eating much nor drinking. She just won't be told!

23 March   Gretel translated a letter from Maria's brother. He will help financially at first in a limited way with the nursing costs and thanked me for all I was doing . . . Maria was cheerful when I arrived, but suddenly had a long crying spell, followed by another fierce attack on my shawl, forcing out stitches with a pencil. I don't know what was behind this outburst – pain, anxiety, homesickness, frustration, boredom?

25 March   A hectic morning. Anna phoned to say she'll be all right for the first week of Maria's return. The warden called to see if he could help. Phoned potential visitors.

I continued to visit Maria daily, and cleaned her flat and made all the arrangements and preparations for her return home.

7. 1 April to 31 July 1985

1 April 1985 D– (or rather, M–) day. Anna arrived with necessary medical equipment and prepared bed. Maria arrived in an ambulance about 3.00. She was restless and attacked me (verbally)! Gretel, who visited, said that Maria was resentful of me, though she couldn't make out why. I think the fact that I was not at the hospital (it wasn't allowed) may have had something to do with it.

She got on reasonably well with Anna, whom, of course, she knew from hospital, but this was a new setting. She sat in a chair and talked non-stop.

I've no idea if she realizes the implications of her situation, nor how she will cooperate. I thought it best to leave her with Anna, though she seemed to resent me going. She is quite unreasonable in its literal sense, and normal procedures are no good. She hasn't seemed a bit interested in moving round the flat.

When I went up again, she'd taken her pills, but for the last forty minutes Anna had been trying to get her to move. However, in her most obstinate and talkative mood, she has remained uncooperative until now (8.30) ... We gradually talked her into moving. She was delighted to be in her own bed and looked so happy, and became congenial with Anna ... Almost at once, she dropped off (9.15). It is good the way she seems to have accepted A. in the flat. Interestingly, she hasn't said a thing about her keys, her big brown handbag or her money.

2 April   At 8am Maria was sitting on her bed, half dressed but refusing to put on a skirt and bothered about her catheter. She'd slept well, but Anna had hardly slept at all, just in case ... At 9.00 Anna went to get some equipment and dressing for Maria's heel. I sat with Maria, watching television. The visiting cat came and Maria was pleased to see it. Anna got back about 11.30 and dressed the heel; she's not happy about it. Nor is Maria, and she's on perpetually about the catheter...

The afternoon continued with Anna knitting and Maria getting restless till given a sedative. Anna is very good and gets on well with Maria, though she is so difficult at times, not being clear about anything, changing her mind and taking a long time to cooperate ... But on being put to bed she became much more contented. Anna can't see that there'll be any improvement mentally or with her bladder and that she could go on living for a long time...

Maria likes bed as much as anywhere and I think that she is no longer very interested in life – she hasn't even looked in the kitchen or out of the window, nor bothered about her bag or money; though she did put the chain on her front door.

This lack of interest was a completely new departure from what Maria had been like before that January fall, and it must, I feel, have indicated some special effect of that fall on her dementia, for it was, and remained, so marked.

3 April   Around 7am Anna phoned and asked me to come up. Maria hadn't gone to sleep till midnight and was up on her own by 4.30am ... She got dressed and sat in her chair, but began to feel sick and remained there, looking miserable, for about two hours. She was on about the catheter, a nurse being in the flat and so on. She can be quite impossible to deal with at times, however hard one tries.

Dr Kilner came about 5.15pm. He repeated that she must keep the catheter and have the nurse; otherwise back to hospital. He thinks she'll have to go to a Home. We've also got to work out who looks after her when Anna goes back to hospital by day and also has night duties.

Through Anna's great efforts we now had two more nurses for nights, and three more for the days from 9 to 11am, with an occasional visit in the afternoon to dress Maria's heel. I did the remainder of the days, from 8 to 9am and from 11 till the arrival of the night nurse at around 7.30 or 8.00. These times might vary, but a general pattern was being established. We started a report book, in which details of what had happened, of medication taken and so on were recorded by the nurses and myself. The additional nurses were Olive Newman and Mrs James for the nights and Kate Baxter, Hannah Malcolm and Mrs Croft for the days.

As well as trouble with the heel, soreness began to develop in the sacrum despite careful attention; constipation became a recurring feature in spite of laxatives; and not drinking enough, which led to murky and offensive-smelling urine, remained a continual problem. Her previous pains and causes of physical distress continued; as did her restlessness and confused behaviour, her lack of cooperation over dressing, washing, pill-taking, going to bed and so on. She also was agitated and cried from time to time.

My caring duties, over and above the daily attention to her, involved an immense amount of investigation, correspondence and telephoning to try to obtain grants from charities, acquaintances and others to help pay for the nursing; and of arranging for people to visit her, especially people who could speak German and, too, who could translate into German my letters for Germany, and then translate the replies. This took up all my spare time, and though some of it could be done during the day when Maria was dozing or a nurse or a visitor was with her, most of it had to be done early in the morning or at night. Currently, I was feeling my way over these administrative matters and developing some sort of technique; but they continued virtually unabated for the whole of the two and a half years Maria was at home. There was no option. During this period, too, and for nearly all of the future, Anna was doing an immense amount over and above the considerable actual attendance to Maria, particularly in finding and organizing other nurses and in seeing to the supplies of medication and other necessities.

4 April   Managed nicely with Maria until after lunch when she became restless and, as ever, hating the catheter. However, she showed some spirit in walking unaided, with me holding up the urine bag, to the bathroom, and then looking in the kitchen and doing one or two things there, including, with my help, making coffee. She was very genial with Anna when she returned. She took her into the bedroom to show her photographs and other things in her handbag, which she'd now discovered.

5 April   Anna said that Maria's walking movements were better, but her sore foot, the catheter and her arthritis pains are still debilitating. There is no doubt that she is glad to be at home; and Gretel said that she found her better mentally, understanding more and producing some coherent sentences . . .

9 April   Maria doesn't seem in too good a mood. Mrs Jackson [a German-speaking visitor who had known Maria before] paid a visit and said Maria was as confused as ever. She was shocked by her changed appearance. It is profoundly sad when one thinks of what Maria was, with all her interests and activities, both mental and physical, and what she is now: a virtual non-event as a person for a large part of the time, often suffering and often difficult. I gave her a pill, but she broke it in half and dropped one half between her legs; she then poured half a glass of fruit juice into her coffee and over a chocolate biscuit.

10 April   Got up at 3.45am to carry on with the 'story' of Maria to send to helpful-sounding charities. Left a note for Anna to contact me before she woke Maria, but she came down at once to say – alas! alas! – that Maria had been sitting in the sitting-room chair since yesterday evening, hadn't slept at all, had talked a lot to herself and was very confused. My goodness gracious me! What a situation and what a day to look forward to. To avoid a repetition, I should try to stop her sleeping by day and so being awake all night.

Kate (doing her morning shift) couldn't get Maria to the bathroom or to use the commode. Kate thinks constipation is making her restless. She phoned Anna, who came over, and they got Maria to do her stuff manually, but she didn't like it.

Maria twice got up out of the chair. She found it difficult the first time, but I got her across the room to look out of the window, which was something; and then she sat at the table, which was a new departure, and watered a plant. On the second occasion she moved from one chair to another and then back again. She finally became quieter, enjoying a film on television.

11 April   Got up very early to carry on with a monumental letter to a charity . . . Saw Anna. Maria had bad pain with her heel in the night, so Anna gave her something and she's going to wait till after 9 o'clock to waken her.

Maria has been extraordinarily docile today even when awake, looking out of the window and not seeming to be here . . . Tomorrow may be a difficult day: we have new nurses on, both morning and night, and Maria may not be cooperative.

13 April   How Maria is afflicted and how little I really seem to help her! It is a horrible time, not least the sadness of seeing her having to be a sort of nonentity in her own home. How she must be longing to die.

I wrote that then, but, as will be seen later, it was certainly not all gloom and despondency. There were many cheerful times, and, despite all the undoubted hardnesses and distress, I chiefly remember her smiling, almost mischievous, face; the real charm of some of her childlike actions; the enjoyment of certain expeditions; and, as one nurse described it, 'her cheery self'. All the multiform badness was, of course, truly there, perhaps preponderantly, but it must be stressed that there were also the other better, happier times as well.

16 April   A sad thing is the way she continues to rip things apart or crunch them up. She keeps pulling buttons off what she is wearing or screws up her clothes and pieces of paper. Yesterday she struck a match (box since removed) and held it to her dress. I crushed her pill and put it into her meat, but she used a nail-file instead of a spoon to eat it. She dozed off before eating her dessert, again with the file!

It could sometimes take Maria two or three hours, or even more, to consume food or drink. If things were left by her, they could often be dealt with in bits and pieces; it didn't seem to matter to her if the tea or coffee was cold.

19 April　　The dietitian came, and while I was talking to her, Maria took the stopper off her urine bag, which I didn't notice till later. I couldn't find it. It upset her and she cried. I was nearly very angry. I found it later on the kitchen window shelf.

22 April　　The main difficulty today has been Maria's continual moving from chair to chair and dragging the urine bag after her – at least twelve times – while I was trying to fix her supper. I kept dashing in and out! One surprising feature was that Maria, sitting at a table in a slightly less mobile moment, wrote quite a lot in a sketch book. It looked to be meaningless repetitive letters, but there were several lines, which included what looked like her name, *Ich bin* (I am) and one or two other apparent words.

23 April　　I gave Maria a reasonable breakfast and then a visit to the toilet – quite successful. She wiped her own bottom...
Was horrified to find that Maria, having become aware of her handbag again, was playing about with some money and jewellery that were in it, and has just lost the gold top off a small pin. It's worrying for money and things of value to be at the mercy of her irrational rambles ... Later she became non-stop in and out of chairs, and dragging her urine bag around ... Hannah, who was on for the night, asked me to go up, as Maria wanted me. At times all was cordial, but at times she was awful in her aggressive irrationality. What *is* God's point about senility?

24 April　　Went up to relieve Hannah at 8am. Maria had had a good night, but she cried because she'd 'lost' her money.

However, Hannah knew where it was and we persuaded Maria to put it in her bag and let me lock it away. The gold pin thing also turned up on the top of a jam jar...

Kate came at 9 and found that Maria's lower dentures were missing ... I went up again at 11 o'clock. All was sweetness and light. Maria was showing Kate one of her history books, and has now accepted the urine bag being tied to her leg... She remained in excellent form. She waved to people from the window and went downstairs with Mrs Croft [the other day nurse] and up the path. And the lower dentures were found! ... As soon as Mrs Croft left, Maria wanted to go out again and, blow me down, she walked as far as the bench without too much assistance ... It has been a surprisingly encouraging day and makes the thought of her going into a Home even more unacceptable.

26 April Maria wandered about and complained about her knee. She kept fiddling with the urine bag. Firstly, she took out the stopper so that the contents spilled on the sitting-room floor, which I had to wash. Then she twice wanted it emptied, though there was little in it. Later, in the twinkling of an eye, she undid her heel bandage and took off the padding, and got really angry when I forcibly prevented her from putting her bare heel on the ground. Fortunately, Mrs James was coming for the night within twenty minutes, and she managed to put on a new bandage. She said Maria was very excitable and had cried. When she went out to get something into which to empty the bag, she found that Maria had pulled out the stopper again, and half the contents was on the floor ... At one stage before Mrs James came I had very nearly bashed Maria.

27 April Maria is not as restless as yesterday, but she does so many irrational things: suddenly tears a page out of a book or magazine; stuffs things away under a bed or chair; washes a picture in fruit juice. It's almost heartbreakingly pathetic to see her do all these things and in the middle of it all wearing her smart green hat.

30 April Diana Marshall [a friend] visited, but Maria spent much of the time wandering about. (A pen and a pair of scissors are now missing!) This was followed by a visit from Erika, who couldn't get any sense out of Maria, but thought she was looking and moving better than in hospital ... Thinking of the future, all one can say is that Maria is likely to be more happy, or at any rate less unhappy, here at home than anywhere else.

1 May   Anna and I had a discussion when Maria had gone to sleep. She said that Maria was in great form and very friendly. It was almost as if they were mother and daughter. This is good. Anna has a great liking for her, and if they really can establish such a rapport, it could do Maria much good. To be loved by someone whom she trusts (trust is very important) *and* to love someone could mean a lot to her. It's certainly not possible with me, while all her other friends are too old or not really close enough.

Anna, who was 25, had a lively, outgoing personality, as Maria had had. The other nurses established excellent relations with Maria, but they were mostly that much older than Anna, which in Maria's case made a fundamental difference to the extent of the rapport.

2 May   Mid-afternoon Maria suddenly started to walk down the stairs. I leapt up to accompany her, but after going out of the door, she decided to come back ... A bread knife and two pairs of shoes have now disappeared! ... I found the shoes stuffed into each other on a shelf, but the bread knife is still missing ... About 7pm Maria untied her urine bag and started to fiddle with it. When I remonstrated and tried to fix it, she became obstreperous.

3 May   I must try to be completely patient today. After all, Maria is virtually a baby and has much distress. But it is very hard at times. One mildly amusing thing happened. Maria'd got hold of her top dentures and had been carrying them around in her hand, but I suddenly saw that they were no longer there. So, as per routine, I looked under pillows, cushions, in cupboards, under beds and chairs, but no teeth. Then I saw that she was actually wearing them! This was something that she'd not done for at least three weeks, so the possibility had never occurred to me!

6 May   Shortly after supper – during which she must have changed chairs at least ten times – Maria went into the kitchen and removed the stopper from the urine bag, which was three-quarters full, and the urine flooded the kitchen floor. Well it saved me emptying it! However, I had to clean the floor and disinfect the floorcloth. Ten minutes later the stopper was out again in the sitting-room. I think that this time it had come adrift because she had dragged the bag along the floor. Also, she tends to keep loosening the tapes that tie it to her leg.

7 May   I keep failing to find things – currently missing are an oil can, a breadknife, a pen, a pair of scissors, and now today, a headscarf and earthenware beaker.

11 May   In the course of her wanderings Maria threw a button into the toilet and 'cleaned' half a loaf of bread with the washing-up mop. I regret to say that I can understand how some people can suddenly batter babies.

12 May   After wandering about, Maria had a very good visit to the toilet, the first for five days. She also twice succeeded (if succeeded is a suitable word) in letting the stopper come out of her urine bag again, so that I had to give the carpet an instant wash. Otherwise she was mostly chatty and calm.

13 May   I offered Maria some orange juice, but she poured it into the wastepaper basket and became churlish, refusing to say good night. She was friendliness itself to Hannah when she arrived. It's important to bear in mind that it's not she who is beastly, but the illness.

15 May   Anna brought a toy dog, a white poodle, which she'd had when she was a child. It seems to have been an instant success with Maria, who talked to and fondled it like a child with a doll. I hope it lasts.

18 May When I went up mid-morning, Maria was restless and wandering, and she got hold of some stamps of mine, which she refused to give up. I have a sore throat, which has made me feel tetchy. I got pretty angry with her and shouted at her. Since then, I've just left her alone like a naughty child. However, I rescued the stamps and she became more pleasant. It was wrong of me to shout at her.

19 May My throat is still sore and I feel definitely below par ... Maria is not very well and has signs of a cough. She stayed in bed in the morning. When she got up later, she 'tidied' the sitting-room, which meant that things got scattered around indiscriminately.

25 May I called on Gretel, who'd visited Maria yesterday. She'd found her as mentally confused as ever. Gretel has been very helpful in calling on Maria and in translating things for me. Like everyone else, she says that I must take care of myself and that I am doing a marvellous job. Am I? I wonder.

26 May By and large Maria was very subdued and she cried a little bit. She is in a sorry state. And what a change, even from what she was before her fall in January. She wasn't this almost total baby then. Often to get her to eat, I have to feed her with a spoon and have to be very careful how I present things to her.

As I became more experienced, I found that the presentation of food could make a real difference to its acceptance: it had to look nice and on a nice plate; never too much on a plate at once. After putting food into a small spoon, I would transfer it to another one so that what was handed to her was not dirty underneath. Also, I put the food at the front of the spoon and never filled it quite full. I learned never to rush her over eating; to try to get her to eat when it suited her, rather than when it suited me; and not to worry if she didn't eat at all. The same sort of thing applied to drinks; for example, she would more readily accept certain drinks out of a wine glass than out of anything else. Also, it was important to try to avoid any distraction. If I wanted her to concentrate on eating, it was wise to have the television turned off and to have things that she liked to look at out of reach. If the television was left on, I had to stagger the feeding. She could never do two things at a time. Indeed, sadly, she very often couldn't do one thing at a time.

27 May   By feeding her, I managed to give Maria some breakfast with one pill in it. But she was tearful, and was clearly glad that I was there and that she had my hand to hold. She then dozed off again ... Later in the morning Kate came hurrying down to say there was a foreign man on the phone. It was Maria's son Ludwig. They had quite a conversation. She was very pleased. He and his wife are coming on a visit in September ... When Hannah came for the night, she was greeted happily by Maria, who was more amiable than usual to me when we parted.

2 June   Maria was cheerful first thing, apart from the occasional cough, but she will *not* go out in this wonderful weather. It seems that she just can't be bothered.

3 June   Maria was amiable but she wanted to know where 'the other men' were, including her brother, Johann. She is totally confused. Anna, who was on for the night, contacted me when Maria was asleep. She said Maria had been very good with her. Maria is indeed so good when she is good; and recently she has been like that much more than the opposite (apart from her inevitable mental aberrations). It will be awful if I can't manage to keep her at home.

5 June   On the way back from shopping I met Maria and Kate. They'd walked as far as the warden's house and then back round the gardens. Good.

6 June   Erika called and had a very happy chat with Maria. Later, she told me Maria was no more coherent, but, she felt,

more contentedly resigned to her situation; though she realized
the sadness of it to some extent, she was being brave about it.
Erika believed it was best for Maria to be at home. Maria was not
interested in painting or doing anything much any more; she was
grateful to me for what I did, though she frequently referred to me
by her brother's name. Erika also felt it was good that Maria was as
vague as she was, for it enabled her to accept things better and to
be more cheerful. She also struck Erika as having become a
gentler person.

While I was out of the kitchen Maria wandered in and poured
milk into the kettle, so that when I boiled it, the milk came
flooding through the spout!

9 June   Though all was well, it was a tedious morning. It took a
long time for Maria to show any interest in anything. Then when
I was about to prepare some bread for lunch, she came into the
kitchen and cut part of the loaf into odd shapes, not that it
mattered much, as it's eatable in any shape. She went into the
kitchen a number of times, doing various things, seemingly
intending to be useful. Though its ineffectiveness is sad, it's good
that she has such gumption. Later, she put some of the nuts for the
birds into her tea and I had to watch that she didn't swallow them.

It was necessary to be constantly on the alert for any unexpected
hazard, which could happen in a split second. It was also important
not to leave things lying about that could be damaged or that she
could use in a potentially harmful way.

10 June   Maria was again on the wander and took one of the
eggs out of the shopping in my basket and put it in a little dish. She
then put the dish and the egg in a saucepan and poured coffee over
them. She then took the lot into the sitting-room and put a tissue
in the pan. She surveyed what she had done and didn't like it
when I moved to take the pan away! I think she thinks she is being
helpful and practical. I then went into the kitchen. When I

returned, the egg had been broken and most of the shell and fluid part was in a saucer. But no sign of the yolk. Out of the window? Eaten? Under the sofa?

Later, she cried as deeply unhappily as she has done for some time. It was after looking at a photo of one of her sons. She became distressed, and wandered about from room to room and chair to chair almost non-stop, but I could do nothing except monitor her and offer help. However, she cheered up for a while before supper.

Looking back, I find both the egg and the photo episodes particularly sad. The egg episode seems to have been a courageous and well-meaning effort to do something good and useful, and yet to have been a complete mess, and to have been treated with a sort of unkind rejection by me. As to the photo episode, it was very sad to see the really good person that Maria fundamentally was so truly and unhappily forlorn. But it was a blessing how her moods, however wounding for her at any given moment, could often quickly evaporate. I suppose it was like the way that a baby or child can change.

11 June   Maria is very variable. Yesterday she couldn't stay put in any chair or room. Today she never moved from the one chair … She perked up briefly, watching *Laramie* on television, but she's still in a poor way.

12 June   Read an Alzheimer's Disease Society booklet. Maria's dementia is certainly along 'normal' lines, though in some ways the better qualities of her nature have surfaced at the expense of the opposite, when it is often vice versa.

13 June   I wish I were more knowledgeable about what to do when anything with Maria is not straightforward – do I encourage her to go to the toilet, do I do anything when she feels her stomach as if she had pain, do I prop her up in her chair, make her eat more/less (or try to) and so on? I so often have to do it all by, hopefully, intelligent guesswork.

15 June   Suddenly I felt inexpressibly sad about Maria and cried. The contrast between what she is now and what she was even before January is really quite awful, and when I think of all her vitality, enthusiasm and the many good and kindly and friendly acts of her *good* side – I forget her faults – it is quite heartbreaking. It's like coping every day with the death of someone you love, with no gradual adjusting to it. Every day it's a kind of new death. And she is in so many ways beyond the reach of the help one wants to give.

16 June   There is no time for proper praying to the extent that there once was, though I must confess that it did not then have much apparent effect on her situation. However, I'm sure I've been given strength and outside help. Perhaps she's been given strength too. It must be so. God can't be neglecting her ...

Much to our surprise, Maria, after two refusals, agreed to Anna's suggestion of a drive in her car. She walked quite well to the car, but it took a long time to get her into the front seat. Anna was a model of efficiency, patience and encouragement. We went up Stonebarrow Hill and sat looking at the view. Maria had a friendly conversation with a puppy that Anna borrowed from a car parked alongside. We then went to the sea front, where Anna brought us ice creams. When we got back, it took several minutes and a certain amount of agitation before Maria could manage to get out of the car. Anna continued to be very good at not pressurizing her. A worthwhile trip.

17 June   Maria had photos of her sons out on the table. She kept looking at them and at one stage kissed them. I am sure that some of her crying may have to do with her missing them.

When Hannah arrived for the night and I came down, Maria

was cold to me. Even though I'm used to it and know that it will
be all right in the morning, it is not exactly rewarding after a full
day's attendance, and with never a 'thank you'. But does a baby
thank its mother? . . .

20 June　Maria was agitated about standing up. However, she
wanted to go to the toilet, which was successful, me wiping her
bottom, at which I am now quite good! How she would have
hated it if she were still she . . .

Two ladies from Social Services, who are very anxious to help,
arrived. They feel that sooner or later Maria might have to go into
a Home; and what would happen if I became ill or whatever? I
have to think about what they say, though I've considered it all
already. My instinct is to trust God, who, so far, has enabled things
to be, on balance, so successful. And seeing Maria so cheerful with
them and with Mrs Wright [an excellent home-help] made me
think how awful it would be to run the risk of taking away from
her such measure of happiness as she can have here.

24 June　Kate came down with Maria to go for a walk, Maria
walking quite well. They were away over twenty minutes and I
was delighted to hear they had been into the church and sat there
for a while, and that Maria 'enjoyed' it. The rest of the day
continued splendidly. Maria was chatting and laughing, and
enjoying animals on television. I've also devised a new aid to good
relations and her well-being by making her laugh. This is
achieved by indulging in antics – acting, gesticulating and walking
in odd ways as one would with a child, or indeed like a real comic
doing a routine. So far it's been very helpful.

These antics remained helpful on and off for a considerable time, and
my repertoire increased. It included wearing one or two comic, or
comically arranged, hats, and odd ways of dressing. Just as she could
sometimes cry excessively, Maria could also laugh excessively. It was
nice, though, when this happened.

25 June   Maria had another walk with Kate. Excellent! And it included another visit to the church ... Mrs Harvey from Social Services came to try some occupational therapy with Maria, but she is not an easy subject. I imagine, however, that Mrs H. must often meet with a disappointing response.

26 June   When my back was turned Maria went to the lavatory on her own, undid the bottom tape of her urine bag and wound it tightly round the stopper so that she loosened it and the contents leaked on the floor. You have to watch her like a hawk when she's on the wander. Yesterday I found two sleeping pills under the couch and her lower dentures under the bed. She must have pretended to take the pills the other night when she was restless, but threw them away instead. One should always watch pills go down.

That was not always foolproof. She could seem to have taken the pills but, by accident or design, have retained them aloft, and then at some stage jettisoned them.

28 June   When I went down to pay the milkman, Maria put the chain on the door and despite listening to me and coming twice to the door, it took her ten minutes to realize what was wanted and unchain it. [This chain was, in due course, removed.] She became interested in some pictures that I'd cut out of magazines, which might just lead to some activity for her.

2 July   I found the day very depressing. Maria was all right, but her doing nothing and not responding, and the lack of communication, with no break or visitors, can be devastating at times. The awful waste of time. And then the absolute negativeness of what is happening to her, with no change, except perhaps for the worse, likely in the future. And for how long? Also, the struggle to get money is very tiring. Then, if I get it, I'm stuck here with her, while if I don't, her future is, to my mind, awful ... I've also got a pain in my gums and in my stomach, a headache and a bit of hard skin on the side of my foot, which makes walking painful. WOE is me. [Poor chap!]

5 July   Maria was in very cheerful mood first thing. But alas, it evaporated, and I wasn't in very good form myself. There was nothing unpleasant about it. It was just a routine moribundity on both our parts. There are times when I just can't be a tonic.

8 July   Kate got Maria to have another walk with another sit in the church, and then on the bus-stop bench to look at the traffic. Maria came back looking lively, with a flower in her dress ... After tea, she was very congenial, walking in the garden on her own initiative, looking at the flowers, etc. sensibly and without help. I almost wondered at times if there was anything much wrong with her!

9 July   The day passed satisfactorily and Maria was in great form when Anna came for the night. Indeed, they were mutually sparkling. Honestly, I must do all I can to enable Maria to stay at home. The value of it for her is so great, and the opposite is so fraught with possible unhappiness.

11 July   It is quite impossible for me to get anything of an administrative nature done when I am up with her, unless she's asleep. And even then, there's preparing meals, clearing up, checking and tidying, and almost invariably looking for mislaid things. (I can't find either of her dentures anywhere, though, in the search, I've found a missing pair of scissors.) ... She was not too bad, except for messing up the supper 'agenda' by coming in while I was getting it ready. Later, I kept her quiet with funny 'acting', but I was tired when Anna came for the night.

12 July   We have a new nurse tonight – Sarah Graham. She seemed to be getting on well with Maria when I came down. Just before she arrived Maria had said – to my surprise – that it would be so much nicer if I could stay up there.

13 July All went well with Mrs Graham (Sarah) last night and again this morning . . . When I went up mid-morning Maria was in great form showing old family photos to Anna. *Stop Press*: I've found the long-time missing bread knife! It was tucked away at the back of a cupboard behind some underclothes! . . .

By the time Hannah came for the night Maria was in a curt mood. Earlier, she had been spoiling another of her treasured possessions, a pin cushion.

Such 'vandalism' occurred from time to time. She would pull things apart, cut them up or mess them about in some way. I never stopped her from damaging her belongings if it gave her pleasure or relief. They were her things and if anything improved the 'quality' of her life, unless it was dangerous, it was welcome. In due course, scissors had to be put out of her reach.

14 July Got up at 4am for an hour, writing two letters. Then rested and tried to meditate; not easy when one's mind is on a job. Went up at 7.50. All in order. When Anna came, I started another massive letter to a charity and, on going up again, Maria and Anna were in great form, having looked at photos and tied ribbon in each other's hair. Maria remained OK, but she got a bit withdrawn towards the time Olive was due for the night, until I started being 'funny' so as to put her in a good humour. I will try to do this regularly, for it's not only better for her, but also for the nurses if she's in a friendly mood; though for me it has, at the end of a tiring day, something of the flavour of 'On with the motley'.

15 July Maria was reasonably OK, and showed signs of unusually accurate recollections of people and places in Germany.

17 July Maria was in good form when I went up, but I had more or less to 'tether' her to her chair. She was so wanting to wander . . . She's been generally calm, looking at cards and photographs and enjoying a Danny Kaye film. She remained so very pleasant that I was quite sorry to leave her when Anna came.

18 July   Anna introduced another new nurse, Margaret Lewis, who is coming tonight. She brought her one-year-old son with her, which gave Maria some pleasure. Maria seemed to get on well with Margaret, and was in great form when the pair of them left.

19 July   All went well between Margaret and Maria last night.

21 July   I am developing quite a 'talent' for drawing funny figures to amuse Maria, not to mention new comic gestures and walks! I'm also improving the preparation and serving of meals in a way that is acceptable to her, *and* in introducing medication into it so that this hardly ever fails, provided, of course, that she eats it.

23 July   During the morning Maria shifted things around and cut off some handsome buttons from some of her good clothes. I thought of trying to stop her, but I decided that her enjoyment mattered more ... In the afternoon there was a ring at my door. Maria had come down on her own initiative with Anna and they were pruning the rose bushes. They then went and sat on the bench by the bus stop. Later, Maria laughed at my comic turns and at what was visually humorous on television ...

I found some 'writing' that Maria had done yesterday. It was sad, a pathetic jumble of letters, though it seems to me that she was obviously trying to express something. The only recognizable word was *mit* (with). It was written quite clearly and the i was neatly dotted. There was also *mi* (a preliminary effort?) immediately in front of it.

24 July   Anna phoned down to say that Maria had pulled out the catheter and could I come up and do the breakfast, while she went to the hospital for another catheter. So up I went. Despite the catheter, Maria was in good form. But when Anna went to her car it wouldn't start, so she had to phone for a tow. Meantime she advised me to restrict Maria's intake of fluids in case of retention.

Anna's position is further complicated in that she has to go to a funeral this morning and the hospital wants her this afternoon. It looks as if I shall be stuck with a thirteen-hour day – 8am to 9pm – which will be the earliest that Anna can come from the hospital. The one good thing is that with the catheter out, I don't have to worry about it being pulled out! Nor do I have to empty the bag or get her to try to drink.

The morning went without much trouble, except that things kept getting mislaid. When Maria starts to move things, they can disappear almost before one has gone out of the room … Dr Kilner came in the afternoon. [He never failed to visit Maria every week or respond to any emergency, and Maria responded to his easy manner.] He didn't think the bladder felt too bad and he left a note for Anna to use her discretion about recatheterization.

When Anna came, she decided to do it with the help of Kate, who has come in just for this. All went well.

25 July   Maria had had a good night from 2am onwards, but until then she had been restless, so Anna asked me to try to keep her awake during the day. I tried to do so by making unnecessary noises and leaving the television blaring, but she resolutely dozed off. It suits me, of course, if she's quiet, but it can make it difficult for the nurses if she's too lively in the evening and at night. Also, understandably, Maria can resent being pressurized and not being allowed to doze if she wants to in her own home. One can't win!

27 July   Anna and Margaret gave Maria a good bath and when I went up again, she greeted me with enthusiasm … Sarah breezed in for the night like a breath of spring, and Maria greeted her with a happy smile.

28 July   There was some sort of leak in the new type catheter bag, but I managed to stop it for the time being by adding the top of a ballpoint pen. Maria did some kitchen 'tidying', which actually included cleaning a saucepan properly. [Circumstances can make a very ordinary event seem important!]

30 July   After lunch Maria dozed, occasionally moaning and whimpering, though I don't know why. It went on for about three hours. Sarah came for the night with photos of her little boy to show to Maria. She told me to let her know if there was any emergency while Anna, who has to go to Scotland, is away.

31 July   Went up mid-morning. Kate had tried to get Maria to go for a walk, but 'No'. When Kate had left, Maria, as far as I could interpret, complained about the way these people have to come in instead of leaving her alone to do things.

I talked with Hannah (after she'd got Maria to bed) about euthanasia. We wondered whether it is really right to do so much to keep people like Maria alive when there is no real life left for them. Hospitals and Homes round here are full of such human wrecks. There must be a divine answer. That's really all one can say about it – with trust.

8.   *1 August 1985 to 30 September 1986*

1 August   Well, we've managed to keep Maria at home for four months when initially it was just a three-week trial period. I hope we've (I've) done the right thing in the short and long term context. Anyway, thank God – and I mean that – for what we've managed, and I believe it's right.

Maria was still in bed when I went up. She'd had an agitated night. I gave her breakfast, but I never left her alone or unlooked at for more than thirty seconds or so at a time in case she got up and pulled out the catheter. She was friendly and talked volubly in German. She again seemed to be complaining about the nurses dressing and undressing her like a child.

3 August   When she got up, Maria started to dress herself and was quite congenial. When Donald Jenkins came with some shopping he had done for me, she got up out of her chair and shook his hand ... After tea she enjoyed a German chat with Mrs Jackson, and at the end politely showed her to the door. But she then had one of her irrational spasms. She took the butter out of the fridge and into the sitting-room, where she cut pieces off it with a pair of scissors, and put some on a saucer, some on a tray and some on a spoon. She then wanted to eat a hunk of it. Everything was becoming so messy that I remonstrated with her, whereupon she picked up the spoon containing the butter and hurled it across the room!

5 August   As he has been doing from time to time, Johann sent Maria another bundle of German magazines. She didn't respond and even got rather annoyed when I said that it was nice of him. One never know what goes on in her mind if, alas, it can be called a mind ...

Preparing and serving her meals so as to try to make sure that she eats properly continues to be quite a job. I seem to have to use two or three plates and lots of cutlery. However, it all pays dividends ...

After tea Maria became very cheerful and frequently laughed (some of it was over-reaction). This was chiefly due to one of the new tricks I've devised. One of my old bedroom slippers has a sizeable hole at the big toe and I stick things through it – a pen, a toothbrush, a tube of toothpaste and so on. It looks comic and when she catches sight of it – for I don't draw her attention to it, though I put my foot where she's likely to see it – it amuses her mightily. This paricular item was one of those malleable brushes you use to clean sink pipes. It's a trick that has come in handy, though I don't like to overexcite her.

7 August   When I went up all was in excellent order. Sarah said Maria had been quite lucid. Later, Kate, who had taken her out, said she had walked more quickly and strongly than for some time ... Dr Kilner came and Maria was very chatty with him. He thought she seemed well.

8 August   Mrs Wright produced a nourishing lunch for Maria, as always. Maria was in fine form. She chatted to such an extent that Mrs W. could hardly get away! She reacts to Maria in quite the right way, though she doesn't understand a word of German. Maria also enjoyed nursing the toy dog and enthused over a book about a puppy. Later, she had a good laugh watching a Laurel and Hardy film. As I watched her, I felt again how awful it will be if I can't manage to keep her at home.

16 August   Maria was calm when I went up. She said I was looking very smart. Actually, I'd put on a tie and brushed my hair well. Reason? I felt so depressed that, emulating Charles I putting on a clean shirt before his execution, I decided I should dress in defiance of my depression.

22 August   I persuaded Maria to have a reasonable breakfast, but it was very slow. When I give her a teaspoon with porridge in it, one of three things happens: she'll let me put it in her mouth; she'll take it slowly out of my hand and feed herself; or she'll reject both. I then wait for a minute or two and try again. It's similar with everything – the cup of tea, the bread and honey. It is terribly sad, this wreckage of humanity that senility is.

23 August   Maria seemed very distressed until Hannah came for the night. Hannah made her perk up at once and used soap and water to take two rings off her swollen fingers.

Maria's fingers had recently been affected by arthritis. The rings had at some stage to be discarded, partly because of this, but also because, when the swelling was not there, Maria would fiddle with them and could easily have pulled them off and mislaid them or swallowed them.

2 September   Maria in chattery and wandering form and kept getting in the way when I tried to prepare lunch ... There was a long session in the bedroom during which she showed me things in her wardrobe. Then after a good supper, she kept looking at the same postcards over and over again and saying the same things, which I couldn't understand. When we watched TV, like a child, she wanted to hold my hand for a while (unless, of course, she thought I was a child).

3 September   Ludwig and Helga arrived from Germany at 2.00, and when they left for a while at 4.30 Maria cried. Then at 5.45, as I was preparing supper, she went emphatically down the stairs and we walked, with various rests on seats, including a number of pews in the church, till about 6.40. When we got back, Ludwig and Helga reappeared and there was a happy hour consuming one or two drinks.

4 September   Shortly after the night nurse left, Maria had an attack of diarrhoea. Her underwear had to be removed; and – oh dear, oh dear – the catheter came out in the process. Hannah arrived at 9.00 with her little boy, who was a great success with Maria, and Hannah said she'd leave the catheter out till two nurses were available.

Constipation was as frequent a cause for worry as diarrhoea. This was not only because of its effect on Maria's general well-being, but because of the technical problems it presented. There was the problem of which laxatives to give her (at times different ones had to be tried), and how high the dosage should be from day to day. It was by no means always easy to strike the balance between too much, leading probably to diarrhoea often coupled with incontinence, and too little, so that Maria became constipated, which often necessitated the real distress and unpleasantness for all concerned of suppositories, enemas or manual evacuation. Whenever I went upstairs and saw BWO – bowels well open – in the margin of the nurses' report book, where the bowel situation, good or bad, was always reported, I breathed a sigh of relief. My heart would leap up, like Wordsworth's when he beheld a rainbow; some rainbow. It is also interesting to note that in the earlier days Maria was referred to in the report books as 'the patient', then, after a time, as 'Mrs Ritter' and, finally, as 'Maria'.

Like diarrhoea, incontinence and constipation, problems with the catheter being pulled out, or, more frequently, the urine bag being disturbed, with consequent leakage or spillage of urine, were not infrequent. Cleaning up messes on clothes, furniture and floors, though not a daily occurrence and not always referred to in these extracts, were constant and became a fact of life.

Ludwig and Helga came for a cheerful chat, though Maria tended to potter about. At about 9.00pm Anna arrived. At once her splendid rapport with Maria shone out. I was particularly impressed by it and the more I think of it, the more it seems to me that Maria, helped as she is by the splendid team of nurses and the excellent doctor and home-helps, is as well off as anybody with her dementia and other ailments could be.

5 September   Ludwig and Helga visited, and proposed a trip in his car. Following a deal of *Nein* and *Ja*, Maria agreed and we had an hour's outing, which she enjoyed.

6 September   Ludwig and Helga left in the early evening. I produced my old school cap and Maria wore it. There was laughter and animation!

8 September   After supper Maria became restless and I discovered that she and her skirt were wet. The tube connecting the catheter to the bag had become loose. So I tried to keep her as contented as possible till Anna came. I succeeded quite well, kneeling in front of her as she sat in the chair. We studied each other's hair and ears and so on, and I made a fuss of her. Anna immediately sorted things out and I left them in good humour.

2 October   I feel myself getting more and more protective and defensive on Maria's behalf. She has lately been at times such a trusting, good-natured, well-meaning child.

3 October   She seems glad to see me in the mornings ... One of the snags is her continued reluctance to drink enough, so that often her bladder doesn't get washed out as it should. Sometimes it's impossible to get her to do more than take a few sips.

4 October   A parcel from Ludwig, not yet opened, gave Maria some tearful moments. I'm sure that at times she is on some level more aware of the facts and implications of her situation than one realizes, but that she maintains a brave front, and for the most part is taking things very much as they come.

8 October   Went up 7.50am. Things not too good. Maria had been violent at one stage last night with Hannah, and when the latter had gone, I had a distressing one and a half hours. Maria seemed most upset, crying and trying to tell me things, but I couldn't understand – I think it was probably something to do with last night – and all I could do was try to comfort her and be attentive.

12 October   Maria seems in a way quite a bit older and mentally vaguer today. I showed her some excellent photos I'd taken of her and some of the nurses. She was completely uninterested. She just extracted one of them, folded it in half and brushed it with a wet teaspoon.

24 October   Maria cut up photos of herself and other things that previously she'd kept carefully for years ... Later, Mrs Wright came to give me a break. It was a big success. As usual, she got on very well with Maria and there was much laughter.

This laughter often arose from looking together at scrapbooks that I had made for her or postcards, and playing with things. It would sometimes culminate, on my return, with me cautiously putting my head round the corner of the door and then quickly withdrawing it (with various permutations on that general theme) while Mrs Wright feigned alarm with Maria.

5 November   To my surprise, Maria got up on her own and even largely dressed herself. But after lunch, she was more 'normal', i.e., pottering about, cutting up photos, moving things around, trying to eat a paper tissue after dunking it in tea.

12 November   Returning from shopping, I heard the admirable Kate taking Maria out for a walk. She manages this very well.

When they came back, Maria rang my bell and sat for a time in my sitting-room. She was calm and affable ... Later, she became passive and disinterested; but she then amused herself to some extent with magazines and doodling. And she laughed a lot at various antics of mine.

13 November   Maria was difficult about eating breakfast. It is disheartening when one takes so much trouble and is met with a curt *Nein*. However, she took bits and pieces over the next hour. I shouldn't be put out. It's neither sensible nor fair. Actually, her *Nein* can mean any number of things, such as: 'Not at this moment, but perhaps sooner or later'; 'No, not ever'; 'I don't mind if you have some too'; or even 'Yes'! ...

Kate kindly took Maria and me to her home, where Maria enjoyed the company of the dog and cat. Kate then took me back, as I didn't want to be out when the home-help called, and she and Maria went for a drive. Maria enjoyed it a lot, and it did a lot of good, for it got Maria mobile and on return she did a lot of wandering. It's good for her bottom not to be too static.

16 November   I found it difficult to keep my temper with Maria's uncooperative behaviour over breakfast. She can't help it, of course, her mind being what it is, but it can be so hard and hurtful, and shatteringly unrewarding at times ...

I couldn't manage to get any outflow from her urine bag. And when her legs are crossed, as they nearly always are, I often fail at first to identify the right leg on to which to re-tie the bag. Life is no bed of fragrant roses at present.

17 November   Maria cried bitterly for a while, as she does sometimes. I am sure that it is in realization of the all-round awfulness of her situation. She said once or twice: '*Ich kann nicht mehr*' (I can't any more). It's heartbreaking. It really is a kind of living death, such as we wouldn't inflict on a dog. Fortunately, she does recover to put on a brave front and to forget her plight at times, but...?

18 November   Preparing her bread and butter, etc. is important. It should be cut in little squares with the butter and honey or
whatever not overlapping the sides, so that she can put it easily
into her mouth without becoming sticky, and so that, lacking
dentures, which she refuses to wear, she can eat it...
Sarah arrived and brought her four-month-old daughter.
Maria at once came to life ... After supper, and having been
previously withdrawn, Maria suddenly became lively again,
full of jokes and very friendly. She really is admirable when
she's like that.

19 November   Maria has developed a tendency to pour fruit
juice and tea on books and magazines, and to put things – cards,
buttons, crayons – into her drinks.

22 November   After some hesitation, Maria let me help her up
from her chair and walked (quite briskly) to the toilet. She had
difficulty in sitting down and cried as I held up her skirt and
steered (and slightly forced) her on to the seat. I think this was
more at the indignity of her helplessness than anything else. The
vicar visited; poor man, he was largely at a loss.

24 November   Maria finished her supper with a good deal of
mutual merriment. Shortly before that, Ludwig phoned from
Germany. Maria was delighted when I told her who it was – 'That
is *wunderbar!*' It took her some time to get to the phone, but she
clearly enjoyed the talk.

26 November   Emma Harvey from Social Services arrived to fit
an attachment to the toilet seat to make it higher. Maria cooperated. Mrs Harvey also produced a gadget that enabled one of
Maria's chairs to be raised higher off the ground.
Tea-time was enlivened by a lady from the Family Support
Group, who came with her daughter and the latter's four-month-
old baby. This was a big success with Maria.

The Family Support Group was one of the sources of help whose services I enlisted. I consistently arranged for as many visitors as possible, people from organizations as well as private individuals. They were almost invariably helpful in one way or another, not only to Maria, but to me by providing a relief. Hints on how to 'deal with' her were sometimes necessary.

5 December   Maria can't concentrate for any length of time. At lunch she wandered about between almost every sip or bite; she took a saucepan out of the kitchen and put it on a radiator; she put a clothes brush into a bowl of water; then she went to the rubbish bag and tried to sort it out at the top (all probably a noble effort to tidy and clean). Now she has got hold of my accounts book and is doodling all over it. However, I see that most of it is being done with the wrong end of the pen. Despite all that, she has been very amiable and cooperative, which, in a way, makes it all especially sad.

6 December   Meals-on-wheels lady offered to organize a Christmas lunch for us if no one else did; and Joan Burton *a recent new nurse* hinted the same thing this morning. That makes four offers so far. Very kind.

7 December   Olive came for the night. I've a feeling that Maria might be difficult after sleeping so much today, but I can't bludgeon her awake. Olive's mother, who has recently developed dementia, is not being easy for her, and her father has just fallen off a chair!

8 December   Poignantly, when we were listening to *Songs of Praise*, Maria got up and went to the door; she wanted to go to the church shown in the programme. She was really distressed when I said that it was too late and that the church wasn't here.

9 December   Kate told me that she will cook a chicken for both Maria and me on Christmas Day. She'll bring it up when she's on duty. I accepted gratefully; and there are still four other Christmas lunches in reserve. Such kindness!

16 December   To some extent I dread the future, especially Christmas, if we can't get Maria's bowels regulated ... It's so tiring, trying to keep Maria contented and to respond helpfully *all* the time ...

I'm sure her irrationality is growing. Meals can become a kind of nightmare when she tries to feed herself – food and drink are liable to be spilt on herself or the floor as she idly turns over a spoon with something still in it or when she tries to wipe it on a cloth. Tonight she tried to spoon something out of an empty egg cup and then tried to drink the egg out of the shell. Oh dear!

21 December   We are running out of nightdresses. One on and three soaking and I can't find another! ... The wind is howling outside. A suitable end to this particular week.

23 December   Donald and May Jenkins called with a cyclamen, making the fifth floral tribute that Maria's had. Surprisingly, she rose from her chair to greet them, and when they left she ushered them to the door. She then waved to them when they reached the bottom of the stairs. She moved easily and did it all very graciously. Both physically and 'actually', this was quite unusual for her present state.

24 December   Hannah, who was on for last night, produced a big box of home-made biscuits, and just after she left a neighbour came with a trifle. When Kate came, she brought a Christmas cake. Later, I found chocolate at the foot of the stairs from Diana Marshall!

25 December   Kate brought us her kind lunch, which we both enjoyed, and a liqueur for me. We had a congenial day.

26 December   Maria was so on the go that I didn't have time to do anything. Then when Anna was due to bring Margaret, who has no car, she phoned to say that Margaret had just had an accident and couldn't do the night. Anna couldn't do it either, as she'd put off yesterday's Christmas party to tonight. However she'd come over and get Maria to bed. She was very upset about it … She came and soon got Maria to bed and right off to sleep. Then, after she'd gone, a friend phoned for her – the idiot! This stirred Maria, for I heard her talking. But I've peeped in and she looks quiet. It's now only 9.30, and Anna said she'll look in early in the morning. But what a prospect. Yes, indeed! Maria soon began to be restless. So I went in, as Anna had suggested, to sit by her and pretend to go to sleep myself. She shut her eyes but, blow me down, Anna's friend phoned again. This woke Maria up completely.

I got her to take an orange drink with two tranquillizers, but it made little difference and she wasn't asleep till 6.00am. I stayed with her, holding her hand, trying to soothe her restlessness and ensure that she didn't interfere with the catheter. She talked a lot, and continually sat up or pulled her legs up. She also tried to pick flowers from off her duvet pattern. Main positive incidents were emptying her bag – quite full and with clear urine, which was very good; giving her a biscuit and fruit drink at about 3.00am; and a cup of tea at 5.00. Now at 6.30 she's still asleep, thank God.

I don't feel as tired as I would suppose – the hours just went by. I'm getting used to letting time pass, which brings me to

27 December,   when she's still asleep at 7.10am. May it continue. But when will Anna come? Meantime I've written letters. Anna arrived as promised, and in very kindly mood, at 7.35. Maria was still asleep. Anna was livid with her friend for having phoned, as there were firm instructions never to do so at night in case of waking Maria up, which is just what happened.

This, by the grace of God, was the only time in all the two and a half years that I was left alone with Maria all night. How very lucky in this respect I was compared with many other carers.

6 January 1986   Sarah gave me a reassuring talk about managing to keep Maria at home. She worked in a geriatric hospital and she says that Maria is a standard example of dementia except that she's much more pleasant than most … Maria was as drowsy as yesterday, not holding her head up and not looking at me or anything. But gentle and passive.

7 January   Maria was smiling and lively; and she took breakfast easily. It's an awesome responsibility when someone shows you the sort of absolute trust that she shows in me at present. You feel that anything that is adverse for her is letting her down.

8 January   I had an uplifting glance at yesterday's and today's Psalms – 'Fret not thyself', 'Put your trust in God', 'Ride on because of the word of truth' – but I reflected that although one can easily proclaim 'For Harry and St George', one still has to fight the Battle of Agincourt. The former is relatively easy, but the reality is much harder. So, girding up my loins as it were, I put on slightly smarter clothes than I'd intended to and shaved carefully. This was useful preparation, for since I went up at 7.40am, I haven't been able to write a word till now, 8.40pm. I've been on the go all the time ... However, I've ridden on and Maria is certainly improved today.

9 January   Maria started to wander and her damned underpants started to slip down, so I went around behind her holding them up until I mistakenly loosened them and found them down round her feet. I worked them free again, but only after a while, as she would keep standing on them. However, she was quite nice about it – took it in her stride as it were!

15 January   So far (3.15pm) Maria has been calm and done some crayon colouring, but she hasn't moved ... There is a new problem. She has a sore ear, which has been oozing pus, and Dr Kilner has prescribed something to be taken before food. I hate medication before food, as it nearly always falls on me to try to negotiate it ... The rest of the day continued well, except that Maria would not get up out of her chair and was troublesome over the evening meal, trying to eat it with her fingers or to clean a full spoon on her bib and napkin. But all quite amiable.

18 January   Spent the morning in Exeter buying toys and things that might entertain Maria. I got about ten items, but they were not the sort that you can hold in your hand and play about with, which is what I wanted. There don't seem to be suitable things ... Maria was very subdued and showed no interest in the first two items that I gave to her.

19 January   Maria very amiable. I gave her another of yesterday's purchases – a 'mosaic set' for making patterns. But she tried to eat the pieces. I got very tired in trying to entertain her, which included 'composing' a rather nice song as I vaguely crooned to her. She likes that sort of antic.

25 January   My inability to get Maria to the toilet these days is worrying. She seems to be reaching a stage where she doesn't initiate going, like she sometimes used to do ... One comforting thing about dementia, says Sarah, is that people often don't get worried by things that would have normally upset them.

28 January   Went up mid-morning and was staggered to find no one there, until Kate appeared, having taken Maria for a walk, which included a visit to watch Mrs Marshall's budgerigar. Kate is remarkable in her way ...
Hannah hopes that, for Maria's sake, the home-nursing can go on for as long as possible, though she did hint that hospital might at the moment be more helpful in terms of Maria's physical problems, but, as she agreed, the other factors may outweigh the temporary physical ones.

30 January   I do deplore my frequent lack of entertaining expertise and inability to get any sort of response from her, though that is not uncommon with demented people. But it can be so depressing and so tiring ... She surfaced about 6pm and became a bit more lively as she watched television. Television has been an absolute godsend as far as she is concerned.

1 February   A doll that I bought for Maria has been a great success. She has kept nursing it and tried to give it some of her lunch. But I don't think it will last permanently.

I was quite wrong. The doll remained a source of very considerable pleasure to Maria. I saw it in a local shop and was inspired to buy it, hoping that she might like it. It was perhaps my most successful purchase. It is a charming little doll, which looks very natural and with eyes that opened and shut. I still have it; I couldn't bring myself to throw it away after her death, for it represented, in concrete form, Maria at her best and happiest during her dementia at home.

6 February   Joan came for the morning with her young daughter. Maria was calm in her chair. The young girl had been playing with the toys that I bought. It's good for her to come, as new and younger faces can be better rather than worse for Maria.

10 February   Maria congenial, but not active. At times she does little more than sit and grunt with a sort of neutral 'mm' ... I sorted out some of her things, mostly painting material, which, sadly, she'll never use again, but which she had husbanded so carefully. It makes me want to weep.

After lunch she contentedly looked at a book and laughed at my antics. She then enjoyed a visit to both of us from Mr Coleman ... During the day I asked her if she was comfortable. She promptly said 'Yes'. 'Happy?' She then promptly said 'No'. I wonder how much she does realize of her condition and situation. Some, I am sure, and she puts on a brave face.

19 February   Maria managed some lunch, but it was spread over two hours and she continues to do nothing but doze or gaze at television. All initiative seems to have gone. She was somewhat perverse over supper, but I managed to keep my cool and, after all, if she doesn't want to eat or drink, why should she? She brightened later.

21 February   Went up at 8am. Anna had discovered that Maria's bed was 'awash with faecal fluid'. There was so much of it that the draw-sheet pads had to be disposed of. [By now pads were often inside Maria's clothes and there always were incontinence pads on her chairs and in her bed.]

23 February   I've been worried about Maria possibly sitting or lying in faeces or urine and being in discomfort until she is attended to, though most of the time she is uncomplaining; and the nurses take great care to keep her clean and comfortable, and to protect the sensitive skin on her bottom and thighs. It's a tragedy how someone who has been as intelligent, interesting and active as she has, is now little more than a baby.

24 February   After supper, Maria chatted amiably to the doll. Hannah, who has been abroad, arrived for the night bringing a box of biscuits for Maria, who beamed and said in German, 'Thank you. That's very nice,' almost as if she was normal.

1 March   In the afternoon Maria got out of her chair, walked to the toilet and sat down (no action), then returned to her chair *all on her own*! It's a long time since she's done anything of the sort.

7 March   Mr Coleman came to visit. Maria sat with a crown on her head, made from one of the fitting-together-of-pieces toys that I'd bought. She looked, poor Maria, genuinely crazy. However, it caused much laughter, especially when I played up with funny headgear and bowed to her, and so on.

8 March   Maria was congenial, though she only watched television, talked to the doll, which remains an immense success, and occasionally looked at postcards and pictures in magazines. She is really extraordinarily nice when she's in form.

9 *March*   Maria was very bright, but at lunchtime became overactive in her cheer and chatter. Then she began to doze intermittently and to become her least attractive self: restless, uninterested in anything and a bit snappy. The way she sometimes sits and just looks morose is, when I'm not in a scintillating mood myself, extremely trying. But there it is. It is after all her ill condition and I'm bound to be stale now and again.

10 *March*   Feel dim, being especially concerned about my present staleness in dealing with Maria and 'entertaining' her. And always in the background is worry about her bowels, and about making meals for her, neither of which ever seems to be straightforward. The lack of communication is also upsetting me more than it used to do, and I feel that Maria, despite everything, is getting more and more isolated. What a moan! But that's how I feel this morning. Well, so what? There have been bad patches before and 'the Lord is at hand'. Don't panic. 'With the help of our God, we can leap over the wall.' Think of things actually going well, and damned well leap over the wall...

11 *March*   It is three years ago today that the devil struck his first fatal blow, when Maria had her fall on the beach. Damn the devil and all his works...

All well on going up. Hannah had Maria up, and she took breakfast well, but when Kate came for the morning shift, she became grim not only to her but to me as I left. One has to work very hard at the moment to try to invoke her more pleasant side. I wonder sometimes if all the hassle over Maria is justified. But I suppose it must be. It's benefiting her on the whole, I believe...

After lunch, Maria gradually became more cheerful, and had a long affectionate chat with her doll, cuddling and kissing, and trying to feed it ... She remained pleasant to me. Her barks are often worse than her bites. Before she dozed, I wrote a large part of a lyric. I've done a lot of this while watching her.

Lyrics were often an element of my caring for Maria, and in a way a kind of prayer. The lyric in question represented my thoughts and feelings at the time, which were centred on trying in a sort of 'spiritual' way to boost Maria and to flush her with courage, comfort, hope and endurance. This one went:

> Never mind,
> One day you'll find
> It's all behind;
> Every tear
> And every fear
> Will disappear;
> You weren't made
> To be afraid
> Or disarrayed;
> Just stand fast
> Until at last
> It all is past.

> Every situation must at some time have an end,
> Today may harm and hurt you but tomorrow be a friend!

I think that was about as far as I got at the time, the singing and lyric being, as it were, talking to her. Later, as I pottered about doing things or watching her doze, I added to it:

> Don't give way,
> Don't let dismay
> Destroy your day;
> Fight your fight
> With all your might
> Till things come right;
> All the while
> Retain your style
> And keep your smile,
> Let your pride

> Stay undenied
> Whate'er betide.

Some have spirits that grow weak when things start going wrong,
But some, like you, have spirits that are destined to be strong.

And so on with, in due course, further verses, ending with:

> Yes indeed,
> My friend, you need
> No other creed
> But never mind,
> One day you'll find
> It's all behind,
> *It's all behind!*

And it became 'all behind'.

Extraordinarily, immediately after I'd copied down those last five
words , I caught the end of a television programme in which a blind
professor recounted how, on being asked by his young son if he
would ever see again, had said, 'No, but I will keep on fighting.' His
son had then said, 'But you won't win.' And he had replied, 'I'll
never win, *but I'll never lose either.*' And, deep down, Maria didn't lose
either.

17 March   Good news. When I went up mid-morning Maria
had had a BO [bowels open] without any laxatives or suppositories. A long time since that has happened. She also helped Kate
to make the bed!

She continued in good form, eating and drinking, and doing
some not entirely vague colouring. But, as so often, she got messy
with it, putting the pencils in the fruit juice, wiping them on her
skirt and getting her hands covered with the colour. Then at
supper, she fiddled about with the spoon and dropped bits of food
on herself. This sort of thing tries me sorely. However, like a
baby, she doesn't think she's doing anything amiss.

18 March   Once more I found Maria very trying at supper.
Instead of eating her mousse, she would insist on smearing it all

over a postcard of a lion cub that I had bought her, presumably either being artistic or feeding the beast. Anyway I was not amused! I can almost understand people battering babies – one can snap after a time.

21 March I went to Dorchester to find more 'toys' for Maria and bought a few things. On my return I found that Anna and Kate had been spring-cleaning, and found one or two 'missing' items. Maria had been in 'tremendous form'.

1 April A year ago today Maria came home from hospital. Little did I expect her still to be at home a year hence. Thank God, indeed . . . She got more and more bored and frustrated, and I felt progressively less cheerful – perhaps it's the antibiotics and pain-killers I have been taking for my teeth.

5 April Father Francis [a priest I knew] called and showed Maria his beautiful golden rosary. Her eyes sparkled. He was concerned about how I was, as well as Maria. He blessed Maria before he left.

6 April After breakfast, Anna arrived and took us to her mother's house for coffee and to play with the dog there. Maria enjoyed it and didn't want to get back into the car. So we continued the visit for another hour. When we then went to the car again, Maria became agitated at the difficulty of getting into it, but it was achieved.

16 April Kate had managed another walk with Maria as far as the church, with a sit there for a while. But Maria was cross at having to leave. I wish I could manage to take her out . . . Most of the day she has not been very lively. There has been little on television, and she has neither eaten nor drunk readily. I am ashamed to say I got slightly sharp at one stage. Also, she was twice somewhat weepy. When this happens I feel very sad, for I don't know why she cries and I can't really help her.

21 April   So far (5.30pm) the day has gone satisfactorily. A new visitor via Social Services, Mrs Gray, stayed for two hours. The idea is that she should relieve me so that I can go out, but I didn't leave today, as people need to be 'broken in'. Maria was in great form playing with the doll and the dog and very chatty. Mrs Gray seems to have the right idea of how to cope and was grateful I had stayed.

29 April   Finished another scrapbook for Maria. I hope it gives her some pleasure, though before long she may tear out the pictures ... She was subdued until I was inspired to 'decorate' the little dog and to talk and walk 'funnily'. She became very cheery and ate a good meal, though she would insist on putting paper, pencils or toys into the various drinks that she has by her side. I think the idea is to make them clean ...

Anna brought Margaret over for the night shift and stayed to have a talk with me. She reaffirmed her concern for Maria should anything happen to me. She is very exercised about it, and would take leave of absence from her job for a time and 'in no way' would she let Maria go into certain Homes.

1 May   All well, though she has not been utterly thrilled with the scrapbook. She quite liked it, especially the pictures of babies, but she was not exactly wild about it. We'll see.

4 May   She is often so irrational. I've just bought her a small porcelain rabbit, but at lunch she picked it up and tried to use it as a spoon: indeed she did so use it awhile ... She looked somewhat askance at the supper I had prepared for her. However, after it had been left beside her for an hour, she decided to eat most of it. And why not such a delay in her own home?

9 May   How I wish Maria could occupy herself and communicate. I tried to figure out forthcoming catering, which is a perpetual bother. And now she is restless, muttering and looking glum; and there is no clue as to what – if, indeed, anything concrete – it is. As a continual assignment this is no picnic . . . She was appalling at teatime and I had to retreat to the kitchen to scream and to hit things, both of which I actually did. I feel nearly overwhelmed with all I've got to do on top of Maria as she is today.

At lunch she played with the chocolate mousse with her fingers, poured the tea into her saucer without drinking it, put toys into the drinks, rammed a biscuit into the mousse; took a spoonful of the mousse and fed it to her bricks, and so on. But the poor thing can't help it. And it's my job. (I apologize to her for my spleen!) Thereafter she improved, and was congenial in her irrationalities. But she must get so bored.

It's been a poor day on the whole. And now it has culminated in Anna phoning at 8.15 (as I was feeling more and more frustrated and peeved) to say that the car that she'd bought today (second-hand) had broken down. Could I lend her the money to pay for a taxi as she had none on her? She added, 'I could cry.' So could I. I must keep my patience working overtime. Maria, too, is getting mutteringly restless. *Quel jour!* Anna arrived at 8.45, taking her disaster in good spirit. I soon came down, but with no heart to do anything. I went to bed having to use dried milk for my night drink – a somewhat fittingly revolting end to a somewhat revolting day.

10 May Maria keeps giving these little moans and rocking to and fro and generally chattering. It's been a distressing day, for this went on all the time; and she seemed really unhappy about something, whether physical or her general situation, I don't know. Moreover she seemed upset because I couldn't understand her. She seems to me to have been, during the last two days, more mentally ill than before. Perhaps it's me . . .

15 May I got up after sleeping well. The sun shone right through my bedroom window and into the hall, where it lit up the face of the Madonna in a picture Maria had painted years ago. I found it a happy, encouraging touch. Maria painted quite a few pictures of the Madonna and Child, all of which showed deep and original overall inspiration, if not being outstanding in the portrayal of faces or hands. I have always regarded them, and her flower pictures, as saying something significant about the real Maria. This is also apparent, strangely enough, in much of her dementia behaviour, which has attracted the nurses and some of her visitors so much...

The weather has been lovely this afternoon. I really wonder if I shall ever be able to go out and about again. And, if so, how and when. Time will tell. Time tells a lot of things.

19 May   Maria, who on the whole had been very unpleasant with me, perked up on seeing Anna coming for the night. Of course she sees too much of me, and she was far from kind when I tried to say good night. So it is.

20 May   Mrs Lever, a possible visitor from The Family Support Group came to reconnoitre. Nice, though she looked slightly nonplussed. However, I think she will give it a try.

22 May   I started breakfast before Joan came at 9.00 to finish it. Joan took her for a walk to her own home nearby, where she met Joan's family. Maria was cheerful with it.

23 May   Mid-morning, Maria was slightly subdued, followed by the frequent mixture of laughing, fiddling and unexplained restlessness and muttering. However, as so often, she suddenly snapped out of it and the afternoon went smoothly, including a twenty-minute visit from the considerate German-speaking and more-than-anybody-but-Mr-Coleman regular-visiting Mrs Jackson. Maria chattered away.

25 May   It takes patient effort to remind myself that this situation is (in some roundabout way) God's script, and that I have got to play my part as well as possible without irritation or anxiety when she moans or whatever. In other words – thinking of

Hollywood – I've got to try to qualify for an Oscar as the best actor in a supporting (literally supporting) role. I must, as necessary, stir myself with the word 'Oscar' (similar to 'Basingstoke' in *Ruddigore*). Maria eventually surfaced and stayed awake with the help of watching *Mutiny on the Bounty* on television. She then had a drawn-out supper, turning down my carefully prepared and generally welcomed dishes. 'Oscar' it was! However, she was amicable.

26 May   Went up at 10.50. The nurse had got Maria up and looking very smart, ready for a trip with Anna in her car at 11.50. Maria got in and out of the car very easily. At lunch she was cheery and in due course ate an omelette. Afterwards we walked about 100 yards to Anna's home and met her mother. It was a good trip.

28 May   Went up 7.50am. Maria was chatting happily to the doll and toy dog, but quite suddenly clouded over and murmured, '*Ich weiss nicht*' (I don't know, or I don't understand), as if she suddenly felt her – as Wilfred Wilson Gibson said – 'heartbreak in the heart of things'.

31 May   Maria was uncheerful and started to doze just before lunchtime. I'm going to let her do exactly what she wants and when she wants, no matter how bizarre, annoying or disruptive – 'Oscar' to the full . . . Later, she became alert and amiable. This was partly, perhaps, because I gave her undivided attention and didn't pressure her in any way or react unfavourably to anything. And I always spoke quietly and slowly.

2 June   Since I took over this morning, Maria's been chattering, incomprehensible and restless, and I've got to weather this, remain patient, and do all the meals until at least 8 o'clock . . .

For the third time, she's poured her drink into a handy toy with a hole in it. The only good thing is that she's drinking a lot; but that means I'll have to empty her bag. All my trust, stamina, hope and patience are needed today. Oscar indeed . . .

Well, Oscar has worked so far (4.30), though the ceaseless

chattering has been trying. However, she hasn't been incontinent, and has eaten well and drunk more than any other day that I
can remember; *much* more. I think I shall have to empty her bag
once more, as it's over half full; a nuisance, as she can tend to resist
me and I feel there's a risk of knocking the bucket over, or of not
closing the stopper properly or of disrupting the connection in
some way. She goes on and on talking all the time.

3 June Found two tablets that Maria had obviously spat out!
... After lunch she became restless and I thought I detected a
smell, so after deliberation, I telephoned an S.O.S. to Joan. I'm
glad I did, because Maria had been incontinent and it was good for
her to be cleaned up. Thereafter she was more relaxed. She
especially enjoyed watching the birds eating nuts outside the
window, and looking at postcards of dogs and cats.

4 June Hannah arrived for the morning with her two-year-
old daughter. Maria smiles so nicely at children ... Later, Hannah
took Maria out for a short walk complete with daughter in pram.

8 June Maria was very subdued and drowsy. Is it the weather
or what? Anna says there does not have to be a special reason: she
has dementia.

9 June I'm glad to say that the scrapbooks I've made have
proved a definite success. Suddenly, after ignoring them, she
enjoys them. And the doll has been a greater source of pleasure
than anything else.

11 June Mrs Gray came at 2.15 and as I write this in the
kitchen I can hear Maria laughing and chatting away, with Mrs G.
doing her audience participation stuff splendidly ... Maria has
been in excellent form, full of fun and good nature.

13 June Maria wouldn't stop chattering. Then she kept drop-
ping things on the floor and pouring her drink into or on this or
that ... She started to weep and moan, and there's nothing one

can do about it. Nor can one understand what she wants or says. No one can have any idea what it's like to cope with this, and also keep up spirits, both mine and hers.

16 June   Kate brought Maria a little Austrian doll. Maria at once enjoyed and talked to it. She's also been very taken with a postcard of a dozing leopard, which was sent to her last autumn. She often sits and gazes at it.

19 June   As soon as today's home-help left Maria became grim and restless, and treated me almost with distaste. This has been something of a new tendency of late. I have to harden myself not to be distressed either by her unhappiness or by the way it is hurtful to me. She must be sick of the sight of me, but I must always remember that such old people can take it out on those who help them most. Perhaps she regards me as a kind of jailer.

22 June   Maria has dozed from 11.30am till now, 4.15. She looked at the tea I brought and then closed her eyes.

What an extraordinary business is this matter of old age, this dwindling of the human mind and body. Why birth, if there has to be death? It's such a fundamental contradiction. Life isn't really life if it dies.

25 June   Spoke on the phone with Mrs Wright. She asked about Maria and said she hoped (as I devoutly do) that Maria dies in her sleep. She said that her mother, who was demented, had had to go to a hospital in the end and had had three terrible months; the old people there were treated like lumps of nothing, just carted about, no dignity or anything. We both felt that for such old people, with no future of any happiness, euthanasia could well be divinely kind. [It was not a local hospital.]

28 June   Maria OK last night but very subdued this morning. Anna thinks it could be because Maria realizes that she (Anna) is in pain. [Anna had injured her shoulder.]

I managed to keep things going. Maria was continually putting bits of the 'stickle brick set' into her drinks. Theoretically, she should never have more than one thing at a time by her, as she is so irrational; but it would be unfair. However, there were some plus items. She really enjoyed an éclair I gave her and she took happy notice of a tea-towel I had bought and put on the back of a chair facing her, a diversion which hitherto she had ignored. She has a habit of coming round to things in due course. The tea-towel showed a picture of two baby fox cubs with their mother.

This was one of several tea-towels I bought or acquired, each showing different animals. Others that I remember were donkeys, an owl, cats – I forget the rest. I changed them daily. Maria didn't always notice them, but they certainly gave her some pleasure from time to time and were worth the investment.

30 June   Maria was very restless and cried off and on. I asked her if she had pain and she replied, '*Uber alles*' (Everywhere), but it's impossible to tell if it is really so, or whether she's just bored, lonely, conscious of her situation or what. When this sort of thing happens, it's damnable. I'm at such a distressed loss and it nearly drives me up the wall when she rocks to and fro and mutters '*Nein*'. Today, in the middle of it all, she stood her doll in a full glass of fruit juice I had just brought her. Dear God, where are you?

4 July   A visitor turned up with a puppy, which was a great success with Maria. She sparkled. Afterwards, she – for the first time in quite a while – got up on her own, and moved to two other chairs and then walked to the bathroom, kitchen and bedroom, where she parked herself on the bed, and we had tea there.

10 July   When Sarah came for the night, I came down pronto, not feeling well. Then, at 10.30 I was sick. Afterwards I sat up in bed and did a crossword, and then tried to sleep. It didn't work and I had a headache. So I am now up at 1.10 writing this and taking aspirin. What an awful day! I'll have to go slow over food tomorrow – no, today. (Don't miss our next horrible instalment!)

11 July   Sarah says that there is a virus around. Two people she knows have had the same symptoms as mine. She says I really ought to stay in bed. Yes indeed.

12 July   Anna phoned to say that she is having great difficulty in organizing the necessary nursing cover. I am reaching the stage of just not bothering. As Thornton Wilder said, 'The years will enfold these things' . . .

Maria had a period of very distressed crying. I think that both in quality and quantity it was the worst bout ever. However, when I paid concentrated attention to her, she began to recover and this was helped by (a) her playing with dolls, (b) me bringing in lunch laid out smartly on a tray; and (c) Charlie Chaplin in *The Great Dictator*. She became very cheerful.

14 July   Maria cried and whimpered off and on, though she was amiable when she stopped whimpering. Also she wouldn't eat lunch. Well, it won't go on forever, and it's my assignment; but I wish there was something I could do. If a plate's dirty, you can wash it; but when there's no practical solution to remedying what you don't understand, and to which there may be no practical answer, it's deplorable. Will I have it all explained when I die? I try to remember the Jesuit in the Russian prisons and Oscar, but to be honest, I think I'm pretty feeble at times.

Today when I think of Maria in that state, I still feel its terrible sadness, even though she is dead and it is all past.

15 July   Went up 7.45am. Maria had been very cooperative with Hannah, but there's blood in her urine and now, too, on her pad because of a pile. But she was pleasant . . . She was relaxed after lunch playing in no sort of rational way with the cards, but seemingly contented. I sat and encouraged her. But I suddenly felt sick like a few days ago. Why? I've got hiccups too. It makes it very difficult to cope with and to do things for Maria, no matter what mood she may be in. I want to go alone into a corner, but I've got to hang on for three more hours . . . I survived!

20 July   Returning from a two-day break – the first for a long time – during which Anna had stood in for me, I found that Maria had had a splendid time. They were at Anna's house yesterday and visited a pub where Maria enjoyed watching pool being played, and today they had a picnic on Dartmoor. Maria apparently loved it all hugely, and Anna described her as 'brilliant' and 'ready to eat anything'. She was certainly in excellent form when I went up.

22 July   Mrs Harvey and another lady from Social Services called. They were concerned about my health, and came to tell me of all the possibilities available for daily or longer breaks, with Maria in day centres or hospital wards, at no cost. It was totally sensible and considerate of them, both for Maria and me, but I wonder how well it would work out on the whole for either of us.

1 August   Went to an Alzheimer's Disease Society meeting of those who are looking after sufferers from dementia. We are known in the business as 'carers'. When I returned, Maria had been reasonably cheerful with Mrs Gray and Mrs Wright, who had been jointly holding the fort.

5 August   It was suggested yesterday that to make more room, I should get rid of some of Maria's books, but that I will not do. I want to keep the place more or less as it always was.

11 August   When I went upstairs at 7.45am I was glad to learn that Maria had been very welcoming to Hannah last night . . . but when I went up again mid-morning, I found that she had been a bit fractious . . . However, she was pleasant when a visitor came with her pug puppy. Maria loved it, though the puppy was a perpetual panter on this hot day. She relapsed somewhat when they went, and became almost abusive to me for a time. However, I managed to get her to take a good supper and she became reasonably cheerful. This certainly is a hard job, and not always very rewarding in what it seems to achieve.

14 August Margaret came for the morning shift at 8.30, but had to call me up to get Maria off the bed and into the sitting-room. Maria can be really difficult to move, for she is so strong. Margaret had never seen her quite like it before, and Sarah, too, had a difficult time last night. Maria is clearly having an un-cooperative patch, for she was the same with Mrs Wright yester-day. Probably, it's just a phase. Maybe she resents being managed in her own home, or she doesn't like me going out, or it's a definite turn in her illness . . .

She was obstinate over eating lunch, when I left Mrs Wright to it. However, when I went up later, it was quite different. Maria was in excellent form and continued to be affable, though supper was, as so often, an irritating trial-and-error job. She's completely unpredictable in her moods and in her likes and dislikes.

Most of the sessions with Mrs Wright continued to be happy affairs. Mrs Wright was always good at sharing Maria's enjoyment as together they looked at books, magazines and cards, played with the toys, or talked to the doll or dog. Mrs Wright made Maria laugh by emphasizing what was humorous or cheerful in the pictures. She would do this with suitable expressions or tones of voice, and she concentrated on what she was doing. And, with Mrs Wright's cooperation, that routine gambit of mine of popping my head round the corner of the door never failed.

After supper Maria suddenly became angry at – so far as I could interpret – her treatment (not realizing what they *had* to do) by one or more of the nurses and at me disappearing when they come. I may be wrong, but I think she often feels that my proper place is in her flat and that I desert her. There is no way of getting her to understand the actual facts or, if she did, to remember them.

17 August Oh, how I wish Maria could entertain herself better and not just sit all the time, even though I don't like it when she starts to wander about. But when she mutters '*Nein, nein*', or just closes her eyes in apparent boredom, I feel I'm at fault. Am I? And I wish she could show some appreciation for all that is done for her. But then, in her state, how can she understand? . . . Supper was the usual irritating time with much wasted effort on my part. But if she doesn't want to eat, why should she? To be frustrated is part of my job.

21 August I am unhappy to learn that Joan's family are leaving at the beginning of October, so one of the local emergency nurses will be gone. Also, Anna is going on holiday from 29 September to 15 October. Furthermore, Hannah will be gone before long to have a baby.

22 August Alas, alas, Mrs Wright's been offered and accepted a very good job away from here and so will be coming for only one more week. This is a great blow, though we've been very lucky to have had so much of her. Things are a bit unstuck at the moment with this coming on top of Joan and Hannah disappearing, and Anna going on holiday. Also, Mrs Gray is away for a time, while Mr Coleman is leaving the district. Well, as I've often told others, a bad development can often lead to something better.

27 August Maria has been amiable but dozing. Mrs Wright arrived to make lunch. I shall certainly miss her, and, alas, tomorrow, which is her day for sitting with Maria for two hours so as to give me a break, will be a washout. It seems that home-helps are in short supply and she can't be spared. But it's a real nuisance. It would have been her last sit-in too. She also missed the last two, and Mrs Gray will miss two of her fortnightly sit-ins. It's something of a bad period.

29 August Maria is eating quite well, but I do get tired preparing and serving meals. Not so tired, though, as the Jesuit humping wood or digging trenches in a Siberian labour camp on an empty stomach with no privacy!

The relativity of an event or situation can often be a valuable help and comfort, and in its way can be an important absolute.

1 September   Maria slept more or less all morning, except, to my surprise, when she surfaced to feed herself the meals-on-wheels meat course. After that, she was lively and amiable; and happily she was in a chatty mood when Ludwig and Helga arrived on a short visit from Germany. It was all most friendly and Maria clearly enjoyed it.

2 September   After considerable resistance on Maria's part, Anna and I got her downstairs to Ludwig's car, and though she seemed a bit disgruntled at first, she thoroughly enjoyed it when we got to the Anchor Inn at Sea Town and had a cordial lunch, the proprietors and one of the locals being most helpful. Ludwig and Helga handled her very satisfactorily and on return they brought her upstairs very well.

3 September   A possible additional nurse came along. She knew Maria in hospital eighteen months ago and was amazed at the change (for the better) in her personal manners...
Shortly after Anna had come, Ludwig and Helga arrived and Anna got Maria downstairs and into Ludwig's car surprisingly quickly. We went to Cricket St Thomas, where there were some animals. Maria didn't like the drive – she gets nervous – but once there, despite it being a bit cold, she really enjoyed it. She walked quite a bit and then readily sat in a wheelchair as we looked at the animals. She was just as pleased – if not more so – looking at all the small children, and she enjoyed the restaurant, wolfing down egg sandwiches.

5 September   The day went well, Maria being in chatty form. This included, fortunately, the two hours when Ludwig and Helga came before they returned to Germany. It's good for them to have seen each other and it was excellent that Maria was for the most part in her best form with them.

This was the last time Ludwig and Helga saw Maria alive. Their visits in these latter years had been very worthwhile. It was not easy for them to see her as she was; nor was it easy for them to 'handle' her, for to react to, and deal with, someone with dementia can be very perplexing, until experience gives a guide. Their time together went pleasantly and smoothly, and though there were no striking signs of it on the surface, I am sure that at some level Maria was happy at their visits. I believe, too – though, again, she showed few outward signs of it – that she appreciated and benefited from the presents and magazines that they sent from time to time and the occasional telephone calls that they made. This was also the case with those from her brother and her niece. None of it was meaningless or without significance.

9 September Maria became somewhat bored, but I managed to enliven her a bit by (a) dancing about, (b) building a wall with one of her construction sets, (c) cleaning a saucepan in her presence and (d) vacuuming the sitting-room floor. At times it's agonizing to get her to sparkle, but if I can get her to laugh it makes a big difference. All progressed amiably through supper, and she spent at least an hour looking at two pictures in one of the scrapbooks; one was of a dog, and one of a boy aged about six or seven. She spoke to and smiled at them, and kept stroking their pictures. Actually, she does that sort of thing quite often. It's really charming and quite touching.

11 September No help from any quarter today, but I managed all right. Maria was OK till supper. She then became talkative and, at one stage, almost agitated at some cards with pictures of flowers. She seemed distressed that they were so beautiful.

14 September Maria was pretty dozy, but she perked up at lunchtime and took some interest in one of the new scrapbooks ... When I came down for the night, I had to repair one of the books where she had picked at the pictures, trying to pull them out.

21 September   Anna will soon be away on holiday for nearly four weeks. However, 'the Lord is at hand', a fact which I must not overlook. Maria was in one of her semi-whining states, but she readily took a good lunch which I fed to her. When I knelt in front of her to give it, I called myself *Herr Unten* (Mr Down) and then when I got up I called myself *Herr Oben* (Mr Up), which seemed to tickle her. One has constantly to think of new ploys; and I wish I could discover more new things to amuse her. The trouble is that for ten hours every day (sometimes a bit less, but sometimes more) one needs constant sources of fresh interest, not only of a regular range such as new pictures to look at, or new things to fiddle with, but also of new ranges, at which I haven't so far been too bright – though the cards, dolls, chessmen, my hats, my antics and the scrapbooks have all been successful. But an expensive kaleidoscope and small xylophone met with no response. I wish I could get hold of some dressing-up properties, including false beards and such like.

I suppose I could have done so, even if not locally, and I'm sorry now that I didn't, because I think they would have been helpful. Another successful ploy was to kneel in front of Maria and say, '*Du bist hübsch* (You are pretty), *du bist klug* (you are clever), *du bist schön* (you are beautiful and fine), *du bist tapfer* (you are brave), *du bist gut* (you are good), *du bist WUNDERBAR* (you are WONDERFUL). The order might vary, but never the effect.

24 September   I was 'disjointed', though I didn't let myself get rattled, when Dr Kilner prescribed antibiotic syrup four times a day. Maria doesn't like it and she won't normally take medication from me. And in ten days' time he goes on holiday and then on a course, so he won't visit again for nearly six weeks. That is a nuisance, for he's very good with his weekly visits and it will mean complications over getting prescriptions. He'll also be away during the last week of Anna's holiday. It's been a bit of a shambles recently, but it's stupid to be put out.

25 September I had to clean or tidy sticky books and things that Maria had either ripped about or stuck up with jam. Also to be cleaned were cards that she had put in the meat at lunchtime. At times she doesn't encourage caring concern! . . . She must say *Nein* about a thousand times a day. Like her chattering, it nearly makes me sometimes want to yell 'Shut up'.

27 September Maria was reasonably cheery at lunchtime, but at supper-time I nearly hit her over the head and walked out. She grimly refused to take the antibiotic direct or in the food that I'd prepared as an alternative. Fair enough, but her manner can be a combination of giggle and ungraciousness, which, when you are trying hard, is infuriating. She has no conception, of course, of how hard it is in so many ways, nor of how very lucky she really is in her circumstances. But there are times when I feel like sending her off somewhere and not bothering whether she's happy or not. I really do feel an 'orphan' tonight and at a loss.

28 September Maria was affable, but, because of the antibiotic, I left breakfast for Kate, and I arranged for her to come in this pm to give it again. When I came down I made some custard as something into which I can introduce it at lunch. I know that 'worse things can happen at sea', but the present is a mainly unhappy state for me. By diligent and cunning means I managed to persuade her to eat an egg at lunch, and then the antibiotic secreted in the custard (with cream and strawberries). She also drank some orange juice, but later I found some of it spilt over the postcards laid out on the table. There's been a lot of spillings lately and I have to keep washing or unsticking anything that can be touched.

9. 1 October 1986
to 20 February 1987

The scarcity of available nurses during the day at this time made me feel very vulnerable, and I was finding the situation difficult. The diary continued to be therapeutic, allowing me to release my frustration, anger and occasional self-pity.

1 October 1986 After supper, Maria became extremely distressed. As always, there was no explanation; it may have been a general feeling, for I'm sure she said (in German), 'It's awful to be old.' And it's awful not to know what's wrong with someone or how to help them ... I wonder sometimes if Maria wouldn't be better off in a Home. Perhaps I'm losing my touch and/or stamina; and there's no one to discuss it with in depth.

2 October When I took Maria the lunch that I'd carefully prepared, she wouldn't eat any of it. However, giving the devil a good right hook, I remained calm and gave her other things. It would be nice if she said 'No' more graciously, and also 'Thank you'. I think that her attitude is sometimes partly due to me being polite with and talking to the home-helps, nurses and female visitors. She thinks she's being neglected and/or that I'm carrying on with them.

8 October Shopped warily and had to have a whisky on my return. I'm having to do this, or take pep pills, much too often at present. I'm glad I don't have to have any social life.

9 October Looked at today's Psalms and lessons. 'God is our *hope* and *strength*, a very *present help*.' 'Be *still* and *know* that I am.' 'Go in *peace*.' I went in peace and felt all right without tranquillizers, pep pills or whisky.

12 October   It's time to get back to the front line. To return to it after even the briefest break, even just down here, is not easy; and the breaks, with their glimpses of the things that I have to give up, tend to tantalize and unsettle rather than invigorate me.

13 October   The afternoon continued in normal style, Maria becoming over-chattery but amiable. And she remained so, though she really is crazy, poor thing, and (so) messy – grapes, which one expects to have been eaten, turn up between the pages of a library book or thrust with playing cards into the chess set box given to her to play with. I've had to take away the pawns and castles because she tends to try to eat them.

14 October   Started long-delayed letter to the solicitor about supervising Maria should anything happen to me. Last night Hannah said that her pregnancy is beginning to make it difficult for her to move Maria properly. So this will be her last shift, at least for some time.

19 October   Phoned Mrs Jackson to inquire about her husband. He had been ill and this has recently prevented her making her regular visits. He's OK now, but she's broken her collar-bone, so she still won't be operational for some weeks. Bang goes Mrs Jackson on top of Hannah and the rest. The current succession of upsets has been extraordinary.

20 October   Maria is in very subdued mood, and there's no one available during the day: Anna is ill, Sarah involved in a court case, Kate and Margaret on hospital duty, and Hannah, of course, out of action . . . Kate asked me to try to keep Maria awake during the day, but that is easier said than done; and she mostly dozed. But when Kate came for the night, she soon phoned to say Maria was asleep. That was a relief.

22 October   One wouldn't believe it! Kate has just phoned to say she can't come this morning, as she's been sick all night. I shot upstairs to Margaret and, mercifully, she can stay on for a little while . . . Maria chatters so that I can't think; or she looks miserable and whines, and I don't know if she 'has' or 'hasn't'. And another nine hours to go. And I've got a tentative sore throat. Ah well. Put your trust in God and anticipate that this tyranny will be overpast . . .

23 October   Throat still sore and finding it more difficult than usual to cope with Maria's continued chattering-cum-whining and *nein*ing, not that she (remarkable woman in her way) is unamiable. The rest of today was awful. I continued to feel rotten and Maria chattered non-stop. One bright spot was that when I was getting some supper for Maria, she suddenly walked into the kitchen. She'd got up and done it entirely on her own, and looked round and went back again, things she hasn't done for months.

24 October   Abnormality is rampant. One flounders along on a wing and a prayer. However, to relieve my gloom, Maria remained amiable.

25 October   Anna has organized a new nurse, Delia Shaw . . . All well with Maria except that the urine is showing things wrong with it. I hope we don't have to call a doctor while Dr Kilner is away.

26 October   I'm feeling somewhat better and Maria's urine is apparently not so bad; but how I wish she'd stop talking all the time and that she wouldn't so often sound and look miserable. I wish I had somebody to share the burden with or at least someone to show appreciation . . . Delia Shaw came for her first night. I showed her the ropes.

Delia certainly proved to be an asset. Her speedy arrival to fill the gap left by Hannah seemed to be one more example of how the whole undertaking was blessed.

4 November   Spent some time getting Maria's library books into a fit state to return – replacing torn out pages and date slips, and cleaning pages made dirty by grapes having been pressed between them.

5 November   Delia phoned down at 10.00pm. Medication given, but she can't get Maria out of her chair, so I went up and helped to move her and walk her to the bathroom and to get her undressed and to bed. It needed considerable persuasion and patience. Fortunately, Maria went to sleep at once.

11 November   The day has been amiable. The moon (just over half) is shining clearly and Maria is very pleased with it.

15 November   I had a hard job getting Maria to eat lunch. She seemed awake, but when I took in, first, a boiled egg and, then, ice cream, she dozed off. I got her to eat the ice cream in the end by whipping it in and out of the fridge, seizing moments when she was awake! Feeding can be quite a problem. It's all right to leave certain things next to her, but timing it with anything that needs more or less instant consumption is not always easy.

19 November   Johann phoned from Germany, inquiring after Maria. But she couldn't get to the phone and I don't think she would have talked rationally even if she'd done so. Sad... Dr Kilner, back from his holiday, came and Maria, who has been remarkably amiable all day, chattered away to him. It's good he's back.

20 November   I read a book about cricket at breakfast, but to do anything other than what is related to Maria does tend to disorientate me from full attention to her situation and has to be watched, despite its element of relaxation. That's why I might think twice about going out on parole if I was in prison. Unsettling. [This was a purely personal attitude, which I wouldn't suggest as any sort of rule or guidance for carers.]

21 November   Maria restless and not too bright. Moved, un-usually, on her own from chair to chair, and then messed about with drinks – stuck a glass containing the remains of her fruit juice into the half-empty cup of coffee, then, extracting the glass, poured the remains of the juice into the coffee. She laughed occasionally but mostly sat with her eyes closed... Later – it's been a long, unhappy day – she put the bishop from the chess set into her mouth and seemed about to eat it. I was glad I was there to take it out. Exit chess set, following the exit of many other small things.

26 November   Maria dozed and we had that trying situation when she's more or less asleep and meals-on-wheels and the home-help to serve it both arrive. Do I wake her or not? Problems like this add to the hassle of the job. By loudly vacuum-ing the sitting-room, we got her to stir and she had a little lunch, with perhaps more politeness than enthusiasm.

27 November   A new and inexperienced home-help, though she did her best to give Maria her lunch and to be friendly, did almost everything in the wrong way, so that she was really a home-hindrance rather than a home-help, poor woman. [She was an exception. Most of the home-helps coped well, though in varying degrees, which was commendable, for it wasn't easy.]

30 November   The day sagged along. Maria OK, but nothing stimulating on television, and the same old books, cards and toys must get very boring for her; and we can't, of course, talk properly to each other. Nor can she read or wield a pen or pencil. It's amazing really how she manages to be mostly cheerful.

2 December Anna came to clarify one or two matters with Delia, who was on for the night, and then we had a talk, including a discussion on the situation should anything happen to me. Anna remains adamant that she'd take compassionate leave to ensure that Maria was properly settled. She would really like Maria to stay permanently at home, if, somehow, a day replacement could be found for me.

4 December I woke up between 2.00 and 3.00am and was sick. Feel (3.45) anything but ready for any sort of fray. Dozed till 6.00. Up for a cup of weak tea, wishing someone could care for me today instead of vice versa. Upstairs at 7.30 still feeling a trifle squeamish. All OK, though Maria seemed subdued. Sarah (on for the night) confirmed that, together with Anna, she'd help to work things out for Maria if anything happened to me.

6 December Maria was alternatively tearful and cheerful, but, on the whole, the day went well. I feel *so* sorry for her at times. A recent bother is that, as she now takes no exercise and just sits in a chair, she's growing too fat for her blouses and skirts.

7 December Anna and a friend came to take Maria for a drive. Anna managed to get her dressed, and they then succeeded in walking her slowly to the car. But with her stiff knee it was not possible to get her into the car, though she tried and tried. It was quite sad.

9 December Gretel called with a letter that she had translated into German for me to send to Maria's brother. She chatted a while with Maria, who was very lively, and Gretel said that she was more coherent than usual, producing some complete and rational sentences, though not with any consecutive thinking.

13 December   Maria continued OK, except for indulging in her tendency to pull pictures out of the scrapbooks that I've made. To pull things out or apart is a marked characteristic of her dementia.

16 December   A surprise visit from Mr Deacon, who used to visit her in Lyme hospital. Maria sparkled and she did so, too, with a lady from the Women's Fellowship, who came almost at the same time. Good, though it's a pity when callers coincide.

17 December   All good again. Kate had brought her dog, which Maria liked. She remained in good form when Mrs Gray came. She likes visitors. Mrs Gray brought some mince pies and animal pictures. Olive Newton brought a Christmas cake, but she couldn't stay. Mrs Gray went at 4.30, a bit tired, I think, with her 'entertaining'. Maria *can* be quite tiring.

18 December   Kate decorated the little Christmas tree she'd brought, hung up some of the cards and put coloured lights round the top of the room. It looked really nice and was extraordinarily kind of her. I was glad to see that Maria was pleased with it.

20 December   The post brought parcels for Maria from Germany. Sadly, they have aroused little response. Maria doesn't really understand.

22 December   Maria cheerful but soon became restive. She is without any interest in the cards and parcels to be opened. I've taken off the wrappings, but I'll wait to disgorge the contents till Maria's had lunch . . . The parcels were full of beautifully wrapped little packages, but Maria just wasn't interested. It's sad after so much good will and effort.

I'm sure I can smell incontinence, but what the hell can I do? I can't go bothering Kate today and there's no one else to call in. Edith Bailey called with presents, but Maria couldn't be bothered . . . It's all bloody miserable and Christmas decorations all round the room! We're both just miserable. She's crying and keeps shaking, and now, to add to my bloody misery, she's started tearing pictures out of my carefully prepared scrapbooks. Bloody hell and that's precisely what it is. It's all too much of a bad thing. Bloody December and troublesome Christmas. And I've got so much waiting to be done downstairs. Oh, bloody, bloody hell. She's nearly driven me mad. She went on chattering away and whining and tearing another picture out of the scrapbook and shaking her head miserably, so that I nearly exploded.

It's so hard at times to endure it all with sympathy and patience, which she deserves, and without self-pity. No one knows what it can be like at the end of ten hours in the middle of all this awful Christmas. How I long to be alone for a few days. (And I do keep smelling something.) Anyway the scrapbooks do give her a lot of pleasure in one way or another.

Anna eventually came, after being delayed, and clearly Maria had done something, for she noticed the 'aroma' at once and said she must take her to the toilet. It's been a horrible day not only for me, but also for Maria, sitting in it probably since mid-morning . . . Anna phoned me at 10.00 to reassure me that all was well: a bit of a mess with Maria, but not serious and she was happily in bed. Anna talked very helpfully to me, just what I wanted, a sort of verbal shoulder to cry on, which now and again I feel weak enough to need.

23 December   When I looked at Maria this morning and considered her present state, I reflected on what Anna so wisely said last night: 'It isn't *really* Maria. It's someone else you're looking after.' Meantime there had been an absolutely magnificent sunrise to encourage me . . . Kate produced more things for the Christmas tree. Maria also enjoyed a visit from Erika, who brought another present, and they talked away in German.

24 December   Kate came for the morning, bringing yet something more – a beautiful Christmas cake, which she had made, and a toy elephant! The latter went down well with Maria, as did a small new scrapbook that I've finished. The meals-on-wheels lady came with a bottle of sherry, to give a glass to each of their 'clients'. A nice touch.

25 December　　Christmas Day, but it's just another day as far as I'm concerned. How else? . . . Anna came for the morning with an assortment of presents, including another Christmas pudding! . . . All was well when I went up again. They had opened Anna's presents, which included a bottle of wine and more food. Then Kate came just after 1.00 with her son, bringing two plates of chicken complete with all accessories, Maria's being all nicely mashed up, and a large trifle and two slices of Christmas pudding and more biscuits. We have been overwhelmed with kindness. Maria was very cheerful and remained so till Anna came for the night.

27 December　　Maria was in cracking form when Anna came at 9.00am, and remained so till she dozed after lunch. I came across the Stuart scrapbook which she had so carefully created; what an enormous amount of study she must have done at one time.

During the afternoon Maria, as is so frequently the case unless she is gripped by television, chattered or whined. But she also paid some affectionate attention to pictures of animals. The whining and chattering demands such endurance!

30 December　　Upstairs at 7.45. Margaret said all was well except that the bed had got wet around 6.00, when Maria had called out what sounded to her like 'bitter'—probably *Bitte, bitte* (Please, please) – and was half up. She had been quite amiable about it. She must have fiddled with her catheter connections. It is distressing to think of her – as indeed of any old wreck who has been a person – coming to such straits, and having to say 'Please' like that.

1 January 1987　　Maria's deeply unhappy today. Over and over again she whines and shakes and rocks to and fro and I haven't a clue what it means. If she were a dog, I'm sure I'd have her put down.

3 January   Heard from Hannah. She had a premature boy just before Christmas. All well.

6 January   The home-help says that if this cold spell gets icy, home-helps like her may not risk the trips from Lyme... The afternoon went on all right, but it required patience. Maria had one of those days when she kept putting cards into the fruit juice or tea. I never know whether she's washing or filing them.

9 January   Anna came at 8.00 for the night looking very poorly, with sinus infection and a bad headache. I myself feel too tired to do much. Maria's about the only one who seems to be well.

10 January   Kate's husband has just phoned (7.15am) to say that she has a very bad cold and can't come for the time being. Called Delia at 8.00 and she'll do tonight and tomorrow morning.

Delia remained a constant and willing 'filler-in'. She was perhaps less tied than the others and luckier with her health, but she was, as the Psalm says, 'a very present help in trouble'.

12 January   Maria cheered up when looking at a picture of a baby in one of the scrapbooks and talked to it for an hour... I started checking the temperature. At 3.30 it was −2°C [28°F] outside and will be as low as −9°C [16°F] tonight, so I've been keeping the heating on; the next electricity bill will be electrifying, as they say.

16 January   Went upstairs at 7.35. Maria asleep, and Sarah and I had a talk. She said she was surprised that Maria hadn't deteriorated more in the last year; that if she went into a Home she would probably deteriorate quickly; and that she agreed with me that if Maria were an animal, she would, out of kindness, be put down. She added that doctors did sometimes avoid prolonging life while maintaining maximum possible comfort. I was very relieved to hear that. She also said that final deterioration and death can sometimes happen very suddenly.

I often thought that one would probably ease Maria out of it if she were an animal. However, in retrospect, I do now wonder if that would have been right until the very end. She had many bad and unhappy times, but equally – though she was largely a wreck of her real self – she had many good and happy periods, and was by no means always glum. To put her down would have ignored that positive factor. It could have been a betrayal of her basic good nature, fine spirit, courage and dignity, which, I am convinced, were always there beneath the surface, and, indeed, quite evident at times.

Maria was amiable when I went up again and continued so, but some things are shambolic. Kate isn't better yet, and Delia has just phoned to say that she can't make it tomorrow morning because of road conditions. Sometimes I feel that it's amazing how I keep going. I haven't had a whole day off since the beginning of July. It must surely be God, who kindly overlooks my weak or self-pitying moments.

18 January   Two years ago today Maria had her fatal fall on the icy grass; and we had that traumatic period at Weymouth, Portland and Lyme. Since then we've been here for nearly two years with other hard and difficult times and no end in sight. Despite all of it, I cannot be bitter or uncompassionate towards her when I think of how much she suffered during that period, mentally and emotionally as well as physically, and of how wonderfully brave she then was and has so often been since. And I am very fond of her . . .

All went well till 3.30 when she became restless. She kept slipping forward in her chair in an awkward way, and, blast it, I think I can smell something. Kate comes at 8.00, so only four and a half hours to go! But this sort of situation is a minor hell. Blast these natural functions. They are a staggeringly messy and unsatisfactory method of dealing with what is necessary; and what is the holy 'school solution'? How should I behave and react? Why, when the will is willing, is the wisdom weak? (That, by the way, is not only powerful alliteration, but a fairly pertinent bit of phraseology.)... However, Maria herself remained reasonably cheerful, despite the suspected incontinence and discomfort. And today is far better than those days two years ago.

I often wondered if it might be possible for someone to invent a form of impregnated padding to minimize the acid effect of faeces if someone has to remain sitting in a mess for any length of time; or a device similar to the urine bag for excrement.

19 January   Why do I find it so difficult to have an easeful mind when there's an adverse and hard situation? I can cope with most things that happen to me except physical pain, but I'm not good when others, who mean a lot to me, are in trouble and/or to some extent cut off and alone.

31 January   I wish Maria could find her journey's end... However, when I went up again, she seemed a good deal brighter, and she has enjoyed a china dog which I bought her this morning.

1 February   I looked again at Maria's history scrapbooks and notes. The amount of research they represent remains staggering. It's so sad to think of all that effort – as with anybody – just going down the drain, so to speak, and, too, of her relatively lonely demented exile.

2 February   Looked at the Psalms and Bible. There can be much inspiring, fortifying, nourishing and underpinning in them. Maria is adequately cheerful today, but I do wish we could get her out. However, I can't manage it, and she's got out of the habit... Took more of her things downstairs. There's much that can be thrown away, though by no means all of it and certainly not her good books. I've at last reconciled myself to this sort of selective disposal, for she isn't 'her' any more.

3 February Found more unexpected bits and pieces, including some notes that I'd written to her in the late seventies when she had the row with Miss Barrett. There were also a couple of family items, which one cannot really throw away, however obsolete. They are all too much a part of the 'her' that really mattered.

8 February I woke at 1.50am with a headache. So up for tea and aspirin, and a read of an article in the newspaper, which made me laugh. I rather enjoy this sort of nocturnal self-indulgence, especially when the headache goes quickly...

10 February I feel poorly. However, I can soldier on. But I wish I could do what the nurses can sometimes do when they are not well – just say they can't come in, so can you please arrange for someone else. [This is not to imply that they ever 'malingered'. Quite the opposite.]

To arrange someone else for me all day is virtually imposs-ible... Upstairs at 7.45am. Maria stirred at 8.45 and I got her to drink a cup of tea and eat a bit of a croissant, but I suppose I did something wrong for she clammed up on me. Glared at me and looked sternly at Kate when she came. It's awful to be treated like a piece of dirt, especially when I'm not feeling well. I need great patience not to bash her at times. It's largely her dementia, of course. I'm sure that at times she thinks that we are all being beastly to her.

11 February Feel pretty lousy. I think my cold is just about at its height. I don't relish the day with Maria... The home-help didn't turn up – she's ill. Everyone else can stop going to work when they're ill. I can't. Nor do I have anyone to look after me!

14 February Anna, due to take over from Margaret in the morning, suddenly arrived early at 7.40. Margaret had phoned her to say that Maria was not well in a more than ordinary way. They wonder if it is something to do with a chest infection or urine. If necessary, Anna will call the doctor. This sounds like a possible serious change. I pray only for her comfort and lack of pain. I shopped, after which Anna phoned to say Maria had definitely something on her chest and had been vomiting. I went up. Maria was lying in bed, propped up with her eyes shut, Anna sitting with her and holding her hand. Anna agrees we should try to keep her at home, but hospital may be better for her...

The doctor (one on duty for the weekend) has just been; Maria has to go into hospital. Some obstruction is making her want to vomit, but she's not able to do so. They must find out exactly what it is, as well as the cause of her chest infection. The ambulance came for Maria about 11.00, and Anna went with her to the hospital. I followed them. I found Maria looking comfortable in bed, but more or less crying and it was awful having to leave her. They are going to examine and observe, and Anna and I go back at 5.00. Anna said she really thought Maria was dying this morning and she can't understand how sudden it all is. She'd had what they call Cheyne-Stokes (I thought at first she said chainsmoking) breathing... Kate was fortunately on duty at the hospital...

Five minutes after Anna had left the hospital, Maria suddenly sat up and looked to me to be having a stroke, which Kate also thought. However, it passed off, and the nurse suggested that it was a kind of fit. She was given some medication and injections. I did not like leaving her but she was in good hands.

I didn't know what the outcome would be, for that sudden attack looked terrible, but in the event Maria had a comfortable night. During the next days all the nurses kept in touch with me, anxious to know how Maria was and to offer help. As one of them said, 'You're not alone; you've got all of us girls.' Next day Anna, to her surprise, found Maria sitting up in a chair and reasonably lively.

Thereafter the nurses all visited her at various times. The doctor said he thought something had got twisted in her bowels and that, once her bowel actions were proper, she could probably come home. And so she did on the 20th, when the ambulance brought her back in the early afternoon in time to enjoy a *Lassie* film on TV. The hospital nurse said her recovery was remarkable.

10. *21 February to 12 August 1987*

After Maria's short stay in hospital, she entered a new, and what proved to be final, phase. She was at times quite cheerful and for the most part amiable, but she went into a gradual decline. There was a marked increase in dozing, and often she seemed to have little interest in what was going on around her and in things that used to entertain her; and she had no apparent wish to go out. She also became a somewhat more dependent baby, though a more affectionate one, certainly as far as I was concerned.

A number of additional physical problems developed, all despite careful attention. These included the persistence of a small haemorrhoid and sore sacrum, and, for a time, a sore heel. She had attacks of wind. A vaginal discharge she had recently developed, progressed and eventually became considerable at times. Her stomach became more swollen and she was increasingly heavy and difficult to move. There were, too, the familiar periods of incontinence or constipation. All these things often caused her distress.

Nevertheless, though she continued to have fractious periods, Maria maintained, for the most part, a strange dignity. I think that, despite the dirtiness and indignities of her condition, she was, consciously or at some deeper level, quietly getting ready to die and to do so in a way that was worthy of the inherent courage, good nature and standards of behaviour that lay behind her disordered mind. She was not going out with a whimper. As a *person*, if not *in* the body though *with* that body, she mostly held her head high.

Her deteriorating physical condition meant that more nursing attendance became necessary. Almost regularly now someone had to come during the afternoons to attend to the pile, sacrum and heel, and to monitor her general condition, and suppositories of one sort or another often had to be given. This meant a lot of hard work for me, for though the extra presence of the nurses certainly brought some relief, there were still the many hours, and worries, of attending to her myself, and I had constant – and they were constant – problems in arranging the nurses' increasing duties. Not only were there the additional afternoon and other hours to be catered for, but, for a variety of reasons, the regular hours also became more difficult to keep covered. Further, in order to give me more time for the increased and demanding administration, I needed to enlist more visitors for Maria and to arrange additional home-helping, which Social Services did their best to supply. This extra help did give me more time for administration, and, occasionally, for some additional and needed physical relief, particularly when I had one or two spells of poor health, which included a severe attack of flu in April.

During these five to six months there were times when – perhaps more than at any previous time – I did seriously wonder if Maria wouldn't have been better off in a Home or, perhaps more satisfactorily, permanently in a hospital if that were possible. Such immediate availability of attention in her deteriorating condition was a prime reason for this consideration. A second important factor was that during her recent hospital stay she had responded much more contentedly than in 1985. Moreover, she had shown some pleased interest in what had been going on around her.

Now that she could not entertain herself at all and was, on the whole, more difficult to stimulate and less ready to be interested in anything, I, and Anna too, sometimes wondered if she wouldn't get more pleasure (to such an extent as was now possible for her) in observing the varied life and people in a ward, than in being confined to the more limited and repetitive activities and people in her own home.

There were these valid grounds for considering such a move – I was more doubtful about a Home, though I explored one or two – but, after talking to the nurses and Dr Kilner, I decided that it was better for her overall well-being to remain at home, unless her physical condition became such that this was clearly not so. I was helped to this decision by the fact that my contact with charities, both old and new, continued to make it financially possible.

21 February Upstairs at 7.40am. Maria asleep. Sarah says that things have more or less returned to what they were, and Maria seemed happy to be back in her own bed ... Maria enjoyed the sudden appearance of the window-cleaner at the window. She continued to be amiable. But one needs to stay with her at meals either to feed her or to stop her tilting a cup or a spoon so that the contents are spilled. She forgets what she's doing. Gretel called and surprisingly found Maria more mentally alert than usual. She even gave a rational answer when asked about the hospital, to the effect of 'Yes, I had trouble with my stomach but it's better now.' This was the first rational statement for months; at any rate relevantly rational, because she may be rational in her inner thoughts.

23 February Maria smiles or tries to when she looks at you, but she's not really interested in anything, and her 'usual cheery self', as Anna and Sarah have called it, is not at present with us ... It's too early to tell for certain, but this looks like a new stage of deterioration.

24 February I slept well till 3.30am. Got up for tea. Back to bed 4.30 to 6.00 for some efforts at prayers. It is difficult not to feel anxiety, feebleness, sadness and daily dread. I almost feel inclined to say, 'You give us this day our daily dread', so fraught and battle-tired do I feel. But I must stagger on ... Chiropodist came and did my feet. Maria watched with interest ... Sarah arrived at 8.30 for the night and found her much improved.

Since Maria was definitely entertained at seeing the chiropodist work and had also been interested in watching people knit or make sugar flowers for cakes, I thought the principle of this might be worth following up: getting in visitors who didn't necessarily try to talk to her, but would *do* things that wouldn't waste their time and would be interesting for her to watch. It's a principle that might apply to any patient or group of patients.

25 February   Maria quiet but affable ... Dr Kilner came and gave her a thorough going over – satisfactory, but anything could happen at any time; and he's not going to subject her to a lot of distressing examinations. This is right. The thing is to keep her as comfortable as possible.

28 February   Anna joined Delia, who had been on for the night. I went shopping, and on return heard Maria crying out. It's heartbreaking to hear – probably recatheterization or a supposi- tory. What an awful business it is ... Yes, Maria had had to be recatheterized and have a bladder wash. But she remained in quite good form, except for the piles, which make her sitting very restless ... This evening Maria said 'I believe I shan't live for very long', or at any rate: 'I believe I shan't (or can't) something for very long.'

4 March   Trying to fit in the extra nursing duties is getting complicated and I don't think Maria likes me deserting her, as it were, so much ... Maria was cheered by a visit from Donald Jenkins and, after him, from Gretel. She gets tired more easily now and is really becoming a poor old thing. Margaret came on at 8.00. I was sorry to leave Maria. I feel I ought to stay with her, but people in Homes get left on their own. As somebody said, 'Life is a play with a lousy last act.' It is often the case.

7 March   Maria was somewhat subdued after lunch. She looks at me so oddly at times, almost as if she was wondering who I am and if I can be trusted. And always she says things I can't under- stand. She must really feel very lonely with no communication except with Gretel and other visitors who speak German. What a lot of time, energy and care is being spent on her with what is really such a meagre result except for the prolongation of her dim existence in – perhaps – a slightly less dim way than it would be elsewhere. It's by no means so clearly worthwhile as it used to be.

8 March   St Paul is useful today: 'We that are strong should bear the infirmities of the weak and not please ourselves.'

I had noticed this before and it always helped me. Two extracts from T.S. Eliot did the same: 'For us there is only the trying, the rest is not our business' and 'Undefeated because we have gone on trying'.

15 March   Shortly after Kate had come for the night, she rang down. Maria was on the floor and I had to go and help get her up. As Kate was leading her to the bathroom, her knees had buckled. She was very sleepy and had been incontinent. We had to manhandle her to some extent. She was pretty good about it, though talking like somebody who was drunk. Maria was glad that I was there (so was Kate), and she dropped off as soon as she was in bed. If only she wouldn't wake up.

16 March   The business that took Maria to hospital last month has certainly deteriorated her, though she has not been specially unhappy. In a way she's not deteriorated spiritually in herself, though she's done so mentally and physically. She has been much more affectionate towards me as never quite before, and, as if realizing my help and caring, finding in me a link with her former self, and her best self at that. She has stroked my face in a way not hitherto done, and it meant a lot to her that I was there last night.

This was, of course, very touching and pleasing to me, and it bears out my belief that behind the temporary ugly façade of Alzheimer's is a person, a soul that matters, alive and biding its time.

25 March   At the moment I feel a curious relaxed optimism about the future, for which I must avoid fretful premature bridge-crossing over rivers that may never come. But I must still always plan. One thing that I must do is to stop drinking quite so much whisky. I've been liable to have a slug in the morning and more than one in the evening, which tends at times to lead to head-aches. I should be less feeble.

31 March   I vacuumed the sitting-room, which made Maria laugh a lot.

3 April Maria got on tremendously well with Mrs Walker (Denise), a new home-help. She chatted away with enormous verve – I think about her youth – and they exchanged kisses.

Denise, like Mrs Wright, was a home-help who especially managed to entertain Maria. Mrs Ellis, who also started to home-help about now had a similar way with her and, in addition, got through an extraordinary amount of housework. I feel that we were very well served by the home-helps, though their continuity varied.

1 April An elderly lady from the Women's Fellowship arrived with beautiful pink and white gardenias. Maria kept saying, '*Schön, schön*' (Beautiful, fine).

11 April Woke at 3.00am with the roof of my mouth very sore. Gargled, and had lukewarm tea. Very painful when I swallow. Got up 6.15, but felt I could stay in bed all day. No breakfast, as I also felt sick. I dread today and tomorrow.

Totally unwell. Anna, who was on, kindly promised to stay until noon, and see if she can get someone in for this afternoon. Lay on bed and continued to be terrible. Anna couldn't get anyone and I had to be on till Margaret came at 8.00 ... It was difficult trying to be fair to Maria, who was full of chat, while I felt like dying on my feet. One hell of a day.

This ack, which was diagnosed as due to a current virus, getting to me when I was in a stressed and tired state, carried on with varying severity until 26 April. The nurses and visitors tried to ameliorate things for me, but all the time I had to carry on with Maria as usual – monitor her condition, 'entertain' her, prepare meals, organize the nursing duties and the visitors, check and keep the medical supplies up to date and carry on with correspondence. She, of course, hadn't a clue that I wasn't in adequate shape or there for anything except for her.

13 April I tottered through a bit of porridge and toast with a scrape of butter and weak tea ... If only I had someone with

whom I could share the responsibility for so many things, apart
from the actual doing of so much ... Shopped in the rain and
could scarcely manage it, I felt so feeble. Like the last stages of the
retreat from Moscow.

14 April   I feel very much less than the dust. When I went up
in the morning, Kate, who had stayed as late as she could, insisted
that I rest on the couch. I did my best to 'entertain' Maria from a
distance, but she was not very cheerful. She's really so unhappy at
times and so alone without proper communication. It's very
distressing, but I can do nothing more...

Had a surprise call from another Women's Fellowship lady
with a beautiful nosegay of spring flowers. She talked mostly to
me, which, unfortunately, cut out Maria. Nor was I in my best
social form.

It was inevitable with Maria's state and her lack of English that
people should talk to me, or to anyone else who was present, rather
than to her. However, I never liked it and I tried to prevent it and
steer everyone to concentrate on her. I think the principle of this is
important. People suffering from dementia are not necessarily in-
sensitive or totally unaware; and I feel that it is a sort of slap in the face
to ignore them or to talk (especially about them) as if they weren't
there. It was not deliberate, of course, but automatic and I myself
was guilty of it at times.

19 April   Easter Day. Throat still not good and a repetition of
diarrhoea and vomiting. I don't think I've ever been so consistently ill before. Feel quite rotten. It's bad for Maria when I'm not
well. Lay on the couch and smiled at her, but talking to her, which
she needs, was painful ... Had to clean two faeces stains on her
duvet. The rest of the day went fairly easily; Maria amiable and
eating quite well.

22 April   I'm absolutely fed up to the bloody back teeth. Not
only does Mrs Gray phone to say she can't come for her useful
visit from 2.30 to 4.30 because of a stomach upset, which means

there'll be none of the spare time I'd counted on, but now at 2.30, there's nothing in Maria's blasted urine bag, which means something's amiss up top; and she chatters away; and no one is coming today. Then meals-on-wheels didn't arrive till an hour late. And it's another beautiful day, which adds sadistic insult to injury.

However, Mrs Ellis was excellent again, but Maria's continual chatter or moaning is diabolical, and this urine worry – still nothing in bag – upsets me no end. Why in God's name can't they make catheters that work properly all the time? And most of the people who should visit never seem to do so now. And I have to carry on trying to be a ray of sunshine . . .

Dr Kilner came and was most affable with Maria. And then – praise be – the cavalry came riding up to the relief of the beleaguered garrison! Nurse Wyke, the district nurse, came to bring a pad for Maria's sore heel and, of course, she was able to unkink the catheter tube, take Maria to the bathroom and dry her and change her pants and padding. (She was surprised how well Maria walked.) I cannot think of a more opportune arrival or of a more welcome visitor for a long time. My spirits soared amazingly.

I could probably have learned to do such unkinking myself, but Maria tended to resist if I tried – after all, I wasn't an authoritative and experienced nurse. In addition, I was apprehensive about anything to do with the catheter in case I might end up pulling it out.

26 April   Miss Booth (Linda) joined Anna during the morning. She is a new nurse coming to replace Margaret, who is leaving the district. She came to be shown the ropes. All was excellent and they and Maria got on well with each other. Maria had the lot – catheter change, bladder wash, urine bag changed, hair wash, 'big bath' and BO [bowels open]. Thereafter she mostly dozed . . . I feel much more like myself again.

30 April   Maria mostly dozed till Mrs Lever, a new Family Support Group visitor, arrived. All went well, particularly when Mrs Lever brought in her dog.

1 May   Came down to do some notes for Anna, but in the middle Delia knocked to say that the catheter had come out. I think she'd had to leave Maria momentarily alone on the toilet, which is risky. By heaven's grace I got Anna on the phone and she'll come over. Meantime, Maria is quite lively. But how lucky I got two spare catheters this morning. Anna was over in a flash. Recatheterization was accomplished and Maria had been 'very good'.

4 May   I'm apprehensive about today [a public holiday, which had brought problems in arranging full nursing coverage]. I'll be on the whole day from 10.00 to 8.00, probably with Maria in an uncertain state and with no help over meals.

Apprehension proved to be premature. Maria was affable and with no signs of dirtiness, and I got her to eat a good bit of meals-on-wheels. Then the rest of the day went calmly and without any natural functions' trouble. But, let's face it, I tend to cross too many incontinent bridges before I come to them.

10 May   Anna arrived in the early evening with two friends, and I was delighted when they manoeuvred Maria downstairs and out for a short walk on the path and in the garden. She managed quite well, though she needed much support and didn't always look very happy.

11 May   Maria, though she had a good breakfast, was subdued; and she remained in a moody state, often looking at me with disapproval ... At lunch she refused to eat anything despite my efforts, but she laughed at times and was fairly pleasant when Delia came ... She remained OK with Delia, then dozed until Kate came for the night, when she started to spark again.

12 May   Maria dozed, but brightened up when Denise came to home-help, which included (surprise, surprise) actually getting Maria to do a little colouring with crayons ... Later in the afternoon when Delia left, Maria said 'Good-bye' to her in

English. Then when Gretel visited, Maria was in sparkling form and, in German, gave a thoroughly rational reply to a question. Three good incidents. There's still 'something there' I'm sure.

17 May Found something 'written' by Maria in 1985. It is a long string of meaningless letters, obviously intended for something but totally irrational. She couldn't manage even that now. Thank God she's retained her capacity to laugh and still to be interested occasionally. I sometimes wonder if it wouldn't have been kinder to put her away somewhere and so perhaps let her die earlier. But she might *not* have died, and here she does at least have some things that have some happy meaning for her.

20 May Got up early to work on notes for the nurses. I feel very depressed ... 7.30: something is amiss, for Kate has just arrived to join Anna, who's been on for the night. It must be catheter trouble again. This is impossible. I've just heard Maria cry out, so it must be recatheterization. Poor, poor Maria. What a hell. Anna called me up before she left. It was what I thought and the bed had been wet again. However, I managed to get Maria smiling and to give her bread and marmalade, two cups of tea and a tranquillizer before Kate came back to get her ready for the chiropodist ... Maria survived that too, though with some protest. The chiropodist said that the sore heel was much better. Maria then watched with interest my feet being done. Thereafter she dozed.

24 May Kate had a bad night with Maria, who had gone on chattering till 3.30am. Sarah, as another stop-gap, came at 10.30. She has also agreed to do tonight instead of Kate. What a kettle of fish. The only settled thing these days is an unsettled state.

Kate had come to fill the gap when the previous night's arrangements fell apart. This willing help from her and Sarah was a great blessing: and, as far as circumstances would allow, over these final months, all the nurses cooperated splendidly when there was an emergency. I and Maria were very lucky.

25 May   I laughed more than I've done for some time at a remark on television. John McCallum was referring to the most stupid line he'd ever heard in a film. It was a film around the days of Robin Hood and a man addressing some soldiers said, 'Men of the Middle Ages, march forward. This is the beginning of the Hundred Years War!' It still makes me laugh tonight.

28 May   When Delia was on this morning, I heard a noise and found her and Maria at the top of the stairs. We managed to take Maria very slowly down the stairs and to walk along the front of the building and back. I don't know how much she really liked it, but it's good to get her moving occasionally. [This was the last time Maria got out for a walk.]

29 May   Maria was at her most aggravating over lunch, unpleasantly refusing almost everything. Nor, of course, was she able to explain why she didn't want to eat. It's very difficult at times to keep my temper, even though it is not her fault.

30 May   Maria was at her most irritating, chattering away, semi-abusing me and being as uncooperative over lunch as yesterday. I really do have to submerge myself.

31 May   All went amicably, including lunch being eaten. But later, Maria switched to her most unattractive unintelligible continual chatter and whine, looking at me all the time and not eating her meal or drinking her tea. On these occasions it's very difficult to feel kind. However, she eventually ate most of the food and drank a cup, but the non-stop whiney chattering is enough to make one scream. Poor thing, she's a real lunatic. If she carried on like this in a Home or hospital, somebody would bash her or they'd have to put her in a room on her own. She'd drive everyone up the wall after about ten minutes, let alone several hours. Then suddenly she wanted – most unusually – to move to another chair, which we achieved, though it made normal administration confusing.

Phoned Olive Newman, whose mother is now like Maria, to see if she could do any stop-gap nursing again. She wasn't very happy about her mother's recent stay in a hospital. 'Home is best', she said.

3 June Maria remained fairly affable, but I fall short in not giving her the total attention that short-time visitors can give, though those who do only two hours find even that a bit long!

7 June Maria remained very subdued and tired. I don't know whether she's not very well or if it's what Sarah calls a recharge of batteries day.

11 June The admirable Mrs Lever came at 2.30 with her dog. Maria perked up at once and chattered happily. Mrs L. really achieved something. She has just the right affectionate approach. She says, as so many of them do, that she is getting quite fond of Maria. This is understandable, for the 'warts' that Maria had, have largely disappeared and she can be especially good with someone whom she doesn't see often.

12 June I really do feel exhausted. What a pair of wrecks we are. Like a couple of beached whales.

13 June Delia and I tried but failed to get Maria out for a walk again. It's a sad thought that she may not be able to get downstairs again, unless carried. She then dozed and was quietly amiable. In fact, it was a pleasant afternoon.

16 June Anna phoned to say that she felt too ill to come tonight – could I possibly arrange for someone else? Phoned Sarah and she will step in, though lateish. Luckily, Maria remains amiable.

17 June The chiropodist says that Maria's heel is much better and will now be looked at every other month instead of monthly. Maria was in good form. . . . By and large we are in the middle of a very good spell, Maria being as well and steady all round as at any recent time. If only she could walk down the steps.

18 June   Phoned Hannah to ask if she, having had her baby, could do any duties again. Not at present. But perhaps after September. Very affable ... Continued to wrestle with nurses' duties. One has to keep checking and adjusting.

19 June   All well upstairs in the morning. Sarah says that Homes have great difficulty in getting staff, and the same is true for people getting nursing care for those at home. We are very lucky.

20 June   Maria was somewhat subdued, not eating or drinking much, though, as always of late, mostly affable. She enjoyed a visit from my cousin Jack. On leaving, he kissed her hand, which she likes, and for which she said '*Danke*' (Thank you).

21 June   On Kate's suggestion, as it is a lovely evening, I walked down to the front. The first time I've been down there (apart from twice in a car with Maria) for nearly three years. Quite a few changes. It made me very sad to see all that Maria enjoyed so much but in which she can now have no part. It's like going to a grave.

22 June   Not very satisfactory upstairs in the morning. There'd been more minor wetness and Maria was subdued and sleepy. Kate thinks that despite recent bowel movements she may need a good clear-out. She also says that Maria's getting very difficult to move ...

I went upstairs at 5.10. Linda was inclined to agree with Kate's suggestion of suppositories for a clear-out and a change of catheter. Maria was not very cheery, but she and her 'plumbing' have had to be somewhat 'nurse-handled' recently ... Sarah came for the night and I was rather sad to leave Maria. She doesn't quite understand what's going on, and I feel like a mother deserting a baby, while she, I think, feels that to some extent I am abandoning her.

26 June   Sarah says that Maria could not be better off than she is here, with many changes of face and the big window, out of which she can see trees, birds, cars and so on. You can't *make* old people enthusiastic if they are feeling uninterested or their minds have 'gone'.

27 June   Maria remained awake and amiable, but very quiet. She seems to be getting rather more pathetic and vulnerable of late, even more of a young child who needs looking after.

28 June   Delia agrees with me that Maria has lately become what I described yesterday. She was sleeping but stirred once or twice and smiled; not bright though. Linda came for the morning shift. She, too, thinks Maria has gone downhill, even in the short time that she's been here. It's not pleasant to have to face each day and worry about not her decline, which must happen sometime, but her comfort and peace of mind.

Linda said Maria ate a good breakfast only with a lot of pressing. As she says, Maria can't be bothered herself ... Maria continued amiable, but almost permanently uninterested and dozing. There is no doubt about her comparative lifelessness in the last few days, but thank goodness she seems comfortable ... She became more jovial for a while when I played the fool; but I can't keep it up all day every day.

3 July   After lunch I faced the trying business of seeing no urine in the bag and with nobody coming for at least five hours. Fortunately, there is no smell or sign of wet. Maria smiled quite a bit and then became a trifle restless. I have *no* idea what the restlessness means, and she can't tell me. I just have to sweat it out and hope she's OK or relatively so ... Meantime, I prepared for any possible emergency and phoned Delia to ask her to come early. As is her considerate way, she did so and I stayed while she dealt with Maria. It was a kink in the tube. After it was sorted out, Maria was cheerful .

7 July   Maria, as well as being dozy, showed signs of some distress. The day dragged on unhappily. An outsider can have no idea what it's really like to sit here watching her do nothing but look miserable, and with no communication, particularly, as was the case a little later, when you think she has a headache and she just can't tell you. You ask her something and she says 'Yes'; but you've no idea if she really knows what you're saying. What an impossible task it can be...

Sarah arrived for the night and Maria cheered up on seeing her. Then, as I'd asked her to do, she phoned down at 10.30 with the excellent news that Maria had been very cheerful watching TV and had had the most enormous BO. Clearly, that must have been worrying her. No one can have any idea how relieved that news makes me!

8 July   All was fair when I went up after the morning shift, except for some pinkish discharge, which, when I came to look at it on the pad , was very bloody. Anna (who has been ill and is not yet well enough to do duties) came for a visit and saw it. She thought it was definitely bad and might be giving Maria some pain. She is very anxious to know what Dr Kilner might say...

Dr Kilner came and examined the pad. He said it, in conjunction with the distended stomach, showed that she had a tumour on the uterus, which he had thought for some time. He is not going to subject her to the trauma of an examination; we are to carry on as we are doing. If worse pain comes along, then it will be coped with. The only object is to keep her as comfortable as possible, including, I would say, mentally. He cannot forecast any time scale ... Maria carried on reasonably well, but there's no doubt that she's not what she was on any level and she can look fixedly fed-up at times. Yet her spirit still lets her light up with a smile from time to time.

I phoned Anna to tell her, and then Sarah, who had once

worked on a cancer ward. She said, as Dr Kilner had, that people with massive cancer often don't have pain; while others with small tumours can have bad pain. Also, the rate of growth of a tumour can be very slow in old people.

10 July I had a useful talk with Sarah at night. Maria will not necessarily have pain, and the discharge will be bad only from time to time. The future is impossible to forecast . . . All went well during the day, Maria quiet but pleasant and seeming untroubled.

Delia, on for the night, phoned down to say all was well. Maria had had some supper with good drinking, a good BO and was safely in bed. I thanked her for all her great and willing help. She said that she was only too glad to come and do it all, and added, 'I shall miss her dreadfully when she's not here any more.' Now, wasn't that nice? It shows not only how lucky we have been, but how worthwhile it has been to keep Maria at home.

11 July Delia came down to tell me that though Maria had had a good night and breakfast, she'd had a nasty pain, which had not been helped by mild painkillers. By a stroke of luck she saw Dr Kilner across the road (presumably visiting another patient) and she called him over. He prescribed a stronger painkiller to use if the necessity arose . . . This seems to be a new serious situation, and if pain is going to happen constantly, I may have to reconcile myself to her hospitalization.

12 July Anna came specially to help Kate with the recatheter-ization that has become necessary. She phoned down to say they were having some difficulty and needed something from Lyme hospital. So I've got Mrs Mason to go and fetch it . . . Was called up. The procedure had been successfully completed. The trouble was caused – or so I gathered – by something to do with the tumour and its association with the catheter, and it is likely to remain. However, Maria had had a tranquillizer and one of the new painkillers, so she was pretty relaxed, and dozed.

13 July I find it difficult not to dread every day. Upstairs at 7.45am. Maria much brighter. She even kissed Linda when she left. Kate came on for the morning shift, but when I returned from shopping, she was at the window and wanted me up. The new catheter had come out. We had a hectic time contacting and consulting Linda and Sarah (the only ones 'on tap') about putting it in, and previous treatment like suppositories, and possible times, and advance pills, and getting another of these special catheters.

In the end it was decided to recatheterize this evening with all three nurses helping. Meantime, I got Mr Mason to fetch the required catheter from the hospital. I also liaised with the district nurse just in case. Kate tried, unsuccessfully, to get Maria to have a BO, and I understand from Linda that the presence of the growth could be affecting her bowel action. It might also at some stage actually prevent the insertion of a new catheter, which will make it necessary for Maria to be kept perpetually padded. Oh God, *why* such a state of affairs? Why do you not call a halt to this cruel farce of life? . . . Mrs Lever came with dog and was very nice to Maria. I then sat holding Maria's hand till Linda came. After some sedation, Maria was put to bed. Cheerful until she drowsed off . . .

Delia phoned to ask how Maria was and offered to come in early tomorrow. Anna phoned, feeling somewhat better. She says she has arranged with her boss to be off for a week if Maria should become terminal. She would very much want to be with her at the end and for Maria to be still at home. They all rally round so well.

Maria remained more or less asleep till Sarah and Kate turned up, Linda arriving shortly after. I came downstairs. It seemed awful for Maria to have to be woken up for this business. The whole situation is terrible. Really. The by-products of the concerned help, Maria's spirit and so on have goodness, but her state in itself is diabolical.

I became very fretted and imagined various horrors, as no word came from upstairs for one and a half hours. Then Sarah phoned to say that Maria had accepted the catheter without any trouble and it was draining well. Moreover, she had thoroughly enjoyed having the three of them there playing jokes to some extent and pretending that her medication was a cocktail. The delay had been because Linda had brought some strawberries and cream, and together with the drinks that I'd left for them, they'd had a session and a talk. All very good.

The current diary extracts may again seem to feature bowels, urine and associated matters to an undue extent. The fact is that (as many carers must find) these issues can be a significant cause of real alarm and despondency, as well as of much troublesome, and often dirty, work; such practical work is not, for most carers, I imagine, as severe a trial as the worry and sadness at the real or imagined discomfort and distress of the person they care for, and about.

14 July   Not much joy upstairs. Maria drowsy, in bed, not eating or drinking and, alas, still, it seems, in some pain or distress. She kept pulling up her legs. I don't know what it means. She looks in pain and says, '*Nein, nein*'. It could be wind? . . .

Anna, much better than of late, came for the night and, after Maria was safely in bed, we had a talk. She had prepared some notes for me and questions to ask Dr Kilner. There's no doubt that we are at some sort of terminal stage, but the time factor is uncertain. It may be that Maria will sooner or later have to go into hospital for the sake of her greater comfort and regular attention. The responsibility on me with her at home, though I want that, is awesome and frightening in a way.

15 July   Dr Kilner came and gave Maria a lot of attention. He clarified matters for me, but he can make no prognosis. However, he did say that if a stage was reached when injections were necessary, he'd arrange for Maria to have an injection pump, whatever that is. This pleased Anna, whom I phoned, because it seems to mean that Maria might not need to go into hospital at the end. But what a business it all is and how nice it would be for her if she could just die. Actually, she's been, on the whole, livelier today.

19 July　Maria dozing but congenial. She ate a good lunch but her stomach looks distended. Mrs Lever came and Maria smiled at seeing her. Between us we managed to get Maria out of the chair and walk her to the window for a look out for five minutes. Thereafter she dozed, chattered or said' *Nein, nein, nein*' till Delia came for the night.

20 July　When I went up after the afternoon shift, Maria was not very cheery and she chattered with the, sadly, inevitable unhelpful response from me. I found the evening very depressing. Maria seemed such a pathetic creature and looked at me like a dog looking at a master who is failing it in some way.

21 July　Got up around 5.00am and spent two hours doing a list of nurses' duties till the beginning of September, and trying to coordinate my thoughts about what may be best for Maria. I feel low and floundering...

When Delia came in the afternoon we managed to get Maria on to her bed for an hour. While she was there, Emma Harvey came and we discussed chairs and Maria's bed. We can I think, via this Social Service help, improve arrangements for Maria's comfort... Maria was quite affable and it's been a much better day all told than yesterday.

23 July　Mid-morning Maria was in her worst non-stop chattering, whining, *nein, nein, nein* mood and seemed pretty miserable, poor thing. Also, nothing in her urine bag, so there must be some kink. It's not possible to make her stand up. She goes rigid and I daren't risk trying to pull her up. So I just devoted myself to her, sitting by her side for one and a half hours till Delia came for the afternoon. She soon untangled the catheter tube, so that all was well and we again got Maria on to her bed for a rest... When Delia left, Maria remained chatty, with much whining and *nein*-ing, till Sarah came; I was pretty exhausted by then with trying to alleviate her condition.

25 July　I have just heard that nice Major Cooper has suddenly lost his equally nice wife, who died from angina. It's odd how those, like her, who have good reason and age for living can die, while those like Maria, who have good reason and age for dying, continue to live. No doubt there are reasons somewhere in the divine think tank ... Maria needs more and more attention and does less and less on her own initiative, so being with her is in some ways increasingly taxing. I doubt if I could manage it now without the afternoon breaks.

26 July　Anna introduced Vanessa Morris, who can do some afternoons. She lives near here. Very nice. Anna feels Maria has reached a very demented stage, and she doesn't know how I stand the chattering ... Maria did chatter as much as yesterday but it was much less distressful. She looked at books and TV ... Mrs Lever came for another visit and Maria was in great form. She really is getting more and more childish; it seems hardly possible.

30 July　Early on, I saw Anna's car outside. This was unexpected, so I phoned upstairs. She'd come early because the catheter had come out during the night and a new one was having to be fixed. Catheter problems seem to have been exceptionally recurrent since Maria has been at home again, and certainly as compared with all of the earlier periods. It is becoming appalling for all of us, including Maria, and not least for Anna, who is again not well and is going straight back to bed. Arranged to get two more catheters, because we must have adequate reserves. When will this tyranny be overpast?

Despite everything, the nurses seem convinced that Maria is as happy as she can be, and better off here than elsewhere. She dozed most of the day, but later she started to chatter. She was glad to have me to sit beside her and hold her hand till Sarah came for the night.

31 July　Delia phoned down at 9.45pm to say that Maria was safely in bed and chattering, but that she hadn't been able to walk her to the bathroom and had only just managed to get her to the bedroom. During the last two or three days there have been increasing comments on a decline in her walking, though it was all right this afternoon. It seems to happen only at certain times, but it is a deterioration.

1 *August*   Will we now, or soon, have to think of using the commode and perhaps moving Maria's bed into the sitting-room and/or changing the general routine? This walking business may be partially due to the new anti-pain medication coupled with the recent extended use of tranquillizers, not to mention the humid weather ... Nevertheless, Maria continues to show such spirit and, when she can, affability, mustering smiles and a measure of cheerfulness and politeness.

Anna, on for the morning, called me up. Maria was fast asleep and Anna could hardly move her. She seems drugged and chesty; still no BO (for three days now) and her breathing is erratic. Also, there is an area of broken skin on her sacrum and considerable discharge. It's a bad set-up. I let her sleep. When she woke, she began to talk in a distressed way. So I sat by her and held her hand. But her distress continued and I saw a heel coming out from under the bedclothes and hanging down the wrong way up. On investigation I found that a leg was also nearly out and the other heel was uppermost. She was virtually lying on her stomach. Moreover, the urine bag was absolutely full. No wonder she was distressed. I phoned Sarah and she came quickly. She soon propped Maria up comfortably, emptied the bag and gave her orange juice.

2 *August*   When I went upstairs mid-morning, Maria had had a massive BO, and she had eaten a good breakfast, but Linda hadn't been able to get her into the sitting-room. Maria was awake and chattery, partially affable and laughing, partially whining, but livelier and looking better than yesterday ... Thereafter she alternately dozed and chatted affably. She seemed more relaxed, but she's now, I think, completely irrational. Vanessa speaks German fluently, and she says Maria says nothing sensible.

5 August   In the afternoon Linda got Maria to walk to the bathroom. She feels that Maria has deteriorated a lot in the last week, including some chest and heart trouble, which may be affecting her walking. She thinks that before long it may become necessary for Maria to stay in bed permanently. Dr Kilner, when he came, largely echoed her views. They both said to see what happens in the next few days . . . This looks like the beginning of the end. If it is so, let us hope that she goes before there is too much distress for her.

6 August   Phoned Delia at 8.00am. Maria has had a good night and, when I went up, things were satisfactory. She ate an excellent breakfast and walked quite well to and from the bathroom. Thereafter she was generally affable and chatty, coupled with intermittent dozing.

When the home-help was here, we suddenly had a worrying half hour with Maria alternately crying out and catching her breath, drawing herself in, and shaking in some sort of pain and once murmuring '*Mutter, mutter, mutter*' (Mother, mother, mother), but then laughing. It seemed so bad that I thought of calling the doctor. Instead, I tried Sarah and Linda for advice, but both were out. However, I luckily got Delia to come earlier in the afternoon. That second opinion and moral support was invaluable to me, though by the time she came, Maria seemed to be better. We thought it was probably an attack of gripe. Shortly after that we got her to rest happily on the bed.

Mrs Lever came at 5.45 for a visit. Maria chatted with her and all went well till about 6.30, when there was a recurrence of the gripe(?) trouble. This alarmed Mrs Lever, but she was a godsend. She gave Maria an indigestion tablet, which I'd dissolved in a drink, and Maria then dozed off.

I had continued to be an almost total failure in getting Maria to take any medication or to drink anything. I would crush pills in the food that she was most likely to accept, and although she never detected the pills, she wouldn't always eat the food.

Anna phoned to see how Maria was. I told her what had happened and she said that she was ready to come over whenever necessary. Delia phoned too, and Mr Woodhouse, the warden, who came to fix a light, said we should call on him at any hour (night included) for any help that he could give. I'm lucky, as is Maria, with all these good souls.

9 August   My God, how sad it all is, and how hard it is at times to keep going ... Maria was chatty when I went up in the morning. When Anna came, she found Maria perspiring profusely and gave her a saline bath and attended to the broken skin on her sacrum. She felt Maria was so unwell that she put her to bed on her side, even though she had been quite cheerful...

Linda, on for the night, phoned down at 10.00pm to say she didn't think Maria was at all well: she had a fever and might, with the recent scanty bowel action, have an obstruction.

10 August   I didn't sleep. Got up at 1.15 to have a cup of tea. Back again at 2.30 and up for good at 5.15. There is soon going to be something hard to be faced ... Linda said Maria had had a good night and the sacrum wasn't so bad this morning, but she still had a fever, was breathless when attended to, and looked like a person who is 'obstructing'. She also referred to Maria's belly probably being tender, as she seemed to try to guard it when turned over...

During the day Maria was much more alert and cheerful. When she wasn't chatting, she sat in the chair with her feet up and dozed ... Before Kate came for the night, I found Maria full of fun until she dozed again ... I prepared notes for a meeting of all the nurses tomorrow to appraise the whole situation.

11 August   Upstairs at 9.15 to take over from Kate. All surprisingly admirable. Good night, during which Maria was turned three times. Sacrum looking much better, and a BO, the best for a long time ... Maria chattered away cheerfully. When Delia came in the afternoon, Maria ate the largest meal she's had recently.

As Delia left, Mrs Lever arrived and Maria was very relaxed; they had a good get-together despite the language problem. Mrs

Lever described her as 'bright as a button'. After she left, Maria became a bit distressed. I waited for the nurses to come for their evening conference, and then came down, until I was asked to go up at about 10.00.

The upshot was that Maria's dementia, together with her worsened physical state, including her inability to help herself any longer, is now such that she cannot be given the proper nursing care she needs by one person – therefore two nurses at a time are needed morning and afternoon as an experimental measure, to start tomorrow. This will mean getting hold of extra hands, but as they all want Maria to remain at home, they are willing to pool current resources to give me time to organize the necessary administration and additional staff. It will require a lot of effort and thought on my part. The ultimate alternative will be a Home or hospital.

After they'd gone and she'd got Maria settled, I talked to Anna, who is a real gem in such a situation. It's a good thing that Maria is now so demented that she almost certainly hasn't a clue about her condition. But there is still something there; a soul that pops up.

12 August   I didn't get to bed till after midnight and didn't really sleep to any purpose, so got up at 4.00 to assess the situation. There's no doubt that this is a last-ditch stand for Maria remaining, and in due course dying, at home . . . .

Maria was asleep when I went up at 8.00am. Kate came at 9.00 and we talked a bit about the future. She can't do many double duties for any length of time. She insisted I must not reproach myself if Maria is hospitalized.

Maria had a good breakfast. Later, she sat in a chair dozing and not looking very bright. However, at 12.30 she started to chat and laugh when talked to, and, for the first time in a long time, started to talk to and smile at one of the toy animals. She was asleep when Dr Kilner came and examined her sacrum and tummy. He'd had a talk on the phone with Anna about the nursing problem and he said that Maria must go to hospital, as in her deteriorated

condition it was no longer possible for her to be properly cared for
at home. I couldn't contradict this, but it made me very sad and
for a moment I was tearful . . .

Dr Kilner phoned Lyme hospital and arranged for the ambulance to come in two hours' time. I phoned Kate to come to
prepare Maria, which she did. I also phoned Delia, who was to be
on tonight; she said she'd like to come over anyhow. I phoned all
the nurses to tell them, or to leave messages.

The hospital was quiet and not very occupied: friendly staff
were around. Maria tended to take it in her stride, chatting or
dozing. I think that in her state she will soon accept it as a way of
life. Delia, who came later, thought so too. She brought me
home. As ever, I hated leaving Maria, but I'm sure she'll be treated
kindly and will adjust to her new surroundings. I pray so and that,
though Dr Kilner says she can stay there indefinitely, she won't
last long. On return I phoned various people, but couldn't get
hold of Anna.

So – I think – ends a great effort. But, oh, how sad it is . . . Delia
will take me in to visit Maria tomorrow. Things do happen
suddenly and I'm very tired . . . Sarah phoned. She feels it's
terribly important that all the 'girls' should not regard the work for
Maria as finished, like 'Over to you hospital. Period.' Contact
with the familiar faces should be maintained. She wants to do it for
Maria and for me: 'I am very fond of both of you.' This is exactly
what I'd been thinking: Maria should not be left with any feeling
that she is being deserted.

The Fourth Period

11. *13 August to 4 September 1987*

So Maria left her last home.

Anna was as sorry about the move as I was, but, like me, she couldn't dispute the logic of it. All the nurses kept closely in touch with Maria and ferried me to and from the hospital every day, where I stayed with Maria from about 10am to 8pm, until the end.

13 August   Well, a new era starts . . . Anna, and later both Kate and Sarah, said that it might be possible, with a change of medication and full care, for Maria to go home again, but, realistically, I feel it is doubtful . . .

Phoned the hospital – 'Chattery at first, but a good night' . . . The post brought a beautiful book with pictures of dogs from her brother Johann, which she would have loved, and still might . . . Arranged to phone Ludwig, especially as he and Helga were coming in September . . . Delia came at noon, cooked me some lunch and then took me to the hospital. Maria was fast asleep in a special chair . . . Later, she stirred and I managed to get her to drink a fair bit of soup, the difficulty being to get her sufficiently awake to open her mouth. At intervals she chatted briefly and smiled, and seemed to be relaxed . . . When Sarah came, she was chirpy as ever. Sarah was great with her, and she then took me home. I had calls from Anna, Delia and Kate to get the latest bulletins and to make sure about me having lifts back and forth.

14 August   Sarah took me to the hospital and went in first. All OK. She stayed there briefly while I waited with her two children. When I went in, Maria, in bed, was chatty and smiling, and stayed so for a while, then dozed . . . Delia arrived 7.30 to take me home. Meanwhile the nurses turned Maria, washed her and gave treatment and medication. She looked reasonably cosy when they'd finished.

15 August   Phoned Ludwig. He's coming 13–18 September, but wants to be kept informed . . . Discussed with Anna the pros and cons of trying to get Maria back home. Anna so much wants it, but we think Maria is as well off here as she can be. Kate thinks she looks as if she wouldn't last long, but you can't always tell by her looks . . . Though it was not, I imagine, a final farewell, I was very pleased when I kissed Maria, asleep I thought, on the brow and she opened her eyes, smiled and closed them again. It was unusual on her part and it pleased me a lot, for it was done in a rather special way.

16 August   Dr Kilner thinks it's probably a matter of weeks. Maria's tumour is growing and she will be kept free from pain as far as possible, though not permanently sedated . . . At home, I gathered a number of the toys I'd bought for Maria, with a view to giving them to some children . . .

Talked a lot with Anna about past successful trips with Maria, all of which she felt had made her being at home, with the pleasure she got there, so worthwhile: so sad it couldn't be managed to the end . . . At the hospital Maria was chatty with me for a while, till she dozed off looking comfortable and not really a bit terminal. It's confusing . . . Read some Psalms – 'All *her* fresh springs shall be in thee.'

17 August   Linda phoned and reiterated her offer to ferry me any time. She said she got on very well with Maria and thought a lot of her, though she had nursed her for only a few months.

18 August   Spoke to Sarah on the phone. She says she thinks Dr Kilner and the hospital don't realize how strong Maria really is . . . Anna came to the hospital at 8.30pm. She saw Maria for a bit and they were both at their best with each other. Anna is so upset at Maria not being able to be at home. She feels awful going upstairs and not finding her there. She longs for her to be back again and would try to engineer it if Maria was definitely near the end. She'd come to collect something and absolutely cried her eyes out.

19 August   I wonder if, though I would like it and Anna devoutly wants it, it would be right to have Maria home for the end. Would it now make any difference to her? . . . At the hospital Maria was only semi-dozy and chatted quite a lot, but just towards the end, she completely clammed up. She didn't doze, but just sat staring fixedly ahead.

20 August   More tidying upstairs, including numerous locks and keys still all over the place. Poor Maria must have been partially demented for a long time. There must have been some unrevealed trauma(s) in her life. Now, despite dementia, her intrinsic cheerfulness and niceness seem to have won the day again . . .

At the hospital I got Maria to both eat and drink, but it was a long process – at least forty-five minutes. I had a napkin handy, ready to quell anything that might dribble down her bib, for she has taken to not holding her head up. However, she seems more comfortable. (What a hell of a time birds would have if their youngsters had to be coaxed into opening their beaks, as is now the case with Maria!) . . . The nurse said that Maria is 'very ill', though she doesn't seem too distressed.

22 August   Sorted through some of Maria's books. She had collected more than I'd realized, and her industry over, and interest in, history and painting were extraordinary . . .

It's been the worst day so far (6.40) at the hospital. Head always hanging down and no smile. Couldn't get her to eat or drink. She was in more distress, and I think pain, than on any previous day, though this may be partially due to being too hot in her chair on this warm afternoon . . . Eventually, her distress seemed so much that I rang the alarm bell (the hospital was especially busy), and she became less distressed when put to bed. The staff have been very good ... Delia came 7.30 and Maria raised a smile for her. Although she semi-dozed, her eyes often stayed open. She seemed unaware and wouldn't respond at all, even though her eyes were still open, when we left ... They now give her four injections a day and have stepped up the dose again.

23 August   Maria has certainly been much brighter and less restless than yesterday ... Anna talked to the staff and they say Maria is so strong that she might have a reprieve in general ways, but they are going to increase the injections a little to try to make sure of obviating pain. Painlessness and comfort are all that matter now.

25 August   Did more tidying upstairs. At present I feel that it's wrong if I'm not doing something for her. At the hospital Maria surfaced sufficiently from dozing to have a bit to eat and drink, and she was reasonably alert, smiled and talked once or twice. Dr Kilner said that generally she is slowly going down, but she is comfortable and has settled in well, and they will continue as necessary with increasing injection doses ... Anna is bitterly unhappy at seeing Maria as she is, though she agrees that it's for the best now. But she misses nursing her and their mutual rapport, which was really quite special and touching. She has a photo of her and Maria on her office desk and people are always asking about it.

26 August   Maria was a bit active, talking and laughing now and again, and I got her to have some supper. After that, she got a completely fixed look and made absolutely no movement beyond some rather chesty breathing ... I was very sad at leaving her looking so forlorn with that fixed stare. I'd prefer to stay by her all the time ... Shortly after 11.00pm Anna phoned to say she had phoned the hospital and they said that Maria had deteriorated very much in the last twenty-four hours, and I should phone Ludwig, as she might die quite soon.

27 August   I carried on through the night and forced myself to eat a good breakfast, though it makes me feel a bit sick ... Phoned the hospital. Maria is weaker but rouseable at times, though not much aware. The nurse gives her twenty-four to forty-eight hours. Phoned Ludwig and Helga. They want to be phoned again this evening ... Found Maria a bit less far gone than I'd expected. She even smiled and talked once or twice, but also stared into space a lot.

She raises her arms a lot, and puts up her hands as if reaching for something. Otherwise she keeps her fists clenched. Father Phillips came and said the Service for the Anointing of the Sick. I am to contact him when Maria dies. I'm glad he came. During the afternoon Kate, then Olive, then Linda looked in. Linda thinks Maria could well go on for at least another week. I tend to feel the same ...

They moved Maria to a single room ... Anna came and treated her with great concern, as did Delia. They were very reluctant to leave her ... Learned from Anna and Kate that at this stage, when a patient is both terminal and mostly unconscious, she virtually doesn't eat or drink. There is the danger that she might choke.

28 August   Phoned the hospital: 'Much the same. Could be a few days now.' ... Phoned Father Phillips. He was very helpful about details for the requiem mass and cremation. Like me, he was surprised that she wasn't looking more like being about to die, though he says that at 85 anything can happen.

Anna took me to the hospital and stayed a few minutes. Maria is in a new hammock bed designed to make her more comfortable and to obviate bed sores. She does indeed look supremely comfortable asleep. I've brought a photo of Maria's mother, whom she adored, to put by her ...

While a visitor was with Maria, Sarah took me to her home nearby for beer and a sandwich – a generous and pleasing interlude. I'm being almost swamped with kindness. On return to the hospital, Sarah stayed for a little and did bits and pieces for Maria, such as moistening her lips, altering her position, putting a cold cloth on her forehead – it's a very hot day ... There was a rather distressing hour with Maria crying in some pain from time to time, as the last injection must have been wearing off and I had to do the best I could holding her hand, stroking her and hopefully whispering soothing prayers till the next injection, which soon took peaceful effect...

Sarah says that when it is all over, the family of nurses, for that is what she feels it has become, must all keep in touch ... More and more I feel that this whole enterprise has been blessed in it having been possible and so successful, with the nurses, the help from the charities and now this final chapter at the hospital, which has happened when the hospital nurses are able to give Maria more attention because there are not too many other patients, and they have shown such really kindly interest ... I feel curiously at peace at the moment.

29 August Anna took me in 10.30-ish, and suddenly Maria was in the most touching and wonderful form with her. Coming round, she recognized her, smiled at her, touched and stroked her, and talked (in German) in her best old-time style, calling Anna '*Liebchen*' (darling) and so on. It was quite remarkable. The cherished mother-daughter feeling has now, I feel, got another dimension, with Maria regarding Anna as her mother as well. It was really most moving and Anna was wonderful at it. I only wish Maria could have died in that happy period, which went on remarkably for over an hour, till she began to be conscious of some pain and it was time for another injection.

This was an extraordinarily moving happening. Maria showed no signs of distress. She laughed and smiled so naturally, and she chattered alertly in German as she stroked Anna's cheek. Anna responded, stroking Maria's cheek and hand, and talking back as she always used to do. I just held Maria's other hand and watched with a sort of golden amazement.

As I wrote later, it had 'a sense of Lazarus emerging from his tomb' and it seemed to be a sort of *ave atque vale*, a 'hail and farewell'. But it was a hail and farewell imbued with triumph, as if saying: 'Thank you. All shall be well. We shall meet again.' It was so eloquent, and so remarkably out of keeping with Maria's present condition and situation that it was like sunshine suddenly bursting through a dark cloud. It was extraordinary, and extraordinarily moving and up-lifting. Unforgettable and unforgotten.

(Some months after writing this retrospective comment I visited the hospital and, having to pass by that room, I stopped and went in. There was no one there, and I pictured those moments again clearly and vividly. It was as if there had been some eternal quality about them.)

30 August Phoned the hospital: 'Much the same.' ... Gretel called. She'd phoned Ludwig. He'd said how very grateful he was for what I'd done and was doing for his mother ... At the hospital Anna looked in for fifteen minutes. She was still full of yesterday's shining hour with Maria ... Maria continued sedated, though responding subconsciously to a touch now and again ... The chaplain, who is also a doctor, looked in. He agreed that painless-ness and comfort are all that matter now.

31 August Phoned the hospital. A little lower every day. Occasionally regains consciousness. All as inevitable. But pain, thank God, is being avoided...

The red rose tree on the wall here, which Maria planted some years ago, has chosen this moment to come adrift and to hang down some of its very colourful branches over the path. It is perhaps an appropriate gesture of respect from nature at the approaching death of Maria, who delighted so much in it.

This strange coincidence impressed me very much. It struck me as having a special significance, like that hour with Anna. The tree seemed to me to be gratefully and lovingly saying its own hail and farewell. I am still moved by that thought every year when I watch it blossom afresh. I believe that, in so many things, there is much more than meets the eye.

On going to the hospital I was quite shocked and tearful for a while: Maria looked like a corpse, but alive. However, she seemed less shocking later. She is [such] a poor wreck, such a tragic travesty of her life, of life itself. I stood by her the whole time, holding her hand, moistening her lips and occasionally replying to some weak-voiced remark. It's little enough, but the most I can do . . .

Delia came around 5 o'clock and, almost immediately afterwards, Anna came too. She was first class with Maria and helped to soothe her, especially after an injection at 6.30. Meantime, she insisted that I go out for something to eat while she and Delia stayed with Maria.

1 September   Kate phoned to suggest taking in one of Maria's best nightdresses so that she can eventually end in it when she is dead, rather than 'any old hospital thing'. A good idea . . . Anna took me to the hospital but had to go soon . . . Hannah called in with flowers to see Maria again. She said it would never have been possible to organize and keep on the nurses if they hadn't developed such an affection for Maria. It's remarkable really the impact she has made, with the good real self coming through after dementia took a real hold . . . Nurses came to give her a MacMillan infusion, which means a steady twenty-four-hour flow of injections, and two stayed with her while I had a lunch in the ladies' day room . . .

I don't think Maria will surface to life again, but there are times when she looks, though weak, still oddly 'unfinished' . . . Kate came at 6.00 and stayed for an hour. She said not to forget that she and her husband live near me, and I mustn't hesitate to go there if I want someone.

2 September   Phoned a local official about an idea Anna had to plant a tree on Stonebarrow hill where Maria's ashes will be scattered. It was well received, and I was told whom to contact . . .

Maria was somewhat jumpy and restless. Phoned Anna to tell

her that Maria was more poorly ... One never knows how Maria really is. She seems settled and then becomes apparently agitated, but they say it can be a kind of spontaneous reflex action ...

Everyone is amazed at how strongly she is lasting. The doctors are not able to predict anything. I am assured that she cannot now be in pain or distress, despite any appearances. They think that on some level she can be aware of my presence and that of other visitors.

3 September Phoned the hospital at 6.45. 'Much the same. Perhaps a little weaker, but she's so strong. Could go on for quite a while.' ... Later at the hospital, an auxiliary brought me a cup of coffee. 'She's a very strong lady, isn't she?' she said, looking at Maria. Indeed so ...

Delia came in for a visit. Later, Maria became somewhat restless till at 6.45 they renewed the MacMillan infusion and also gave her a straightforward injection ... She's becoming a bit more poorly all the time: inevitable, of course.

Anna came about 7.15 and was very sad at seeing Maria in her present state, wheezing, jerking her arms, but, as she said, one must think that Maria herself is not upset and can't possibly feel pain with all the injections. She took me home and ventured upstairs to see Maria's flat again, which she'd rather dreaded. She was pleased to see that everything was as it had been before, as if Maria were still in residence, except for the two beds not being made up. And so it will stay till everything is over.

4 September Phoned the hospital: 'Much the same.' Phoned Anna to tell her, and then the others, all full of readiness to help. Did a little sorting upstairs, putting most things back into their previous place, because I agree with Anna that there is something not quite right with disposing of, or rearranging them, till after the funeral. It seems more fitting to leave the flat as if Maria were coming home again. Anna and the others want to arrange a buffet in the flat for everyone after the funeral ...

Maria was peacefully asleep when I went to the hospital at 10.00, but at 11.00 she became a bit restless, so they turned her over and washed her and gave her an additional injection. At about noon I noticed some phlegm coming out of her mouth. I got the nurses to do something about it, and they said that I might as well go and have my lunch. I'd barely started on it when a nurse came and said 'She's gone.'

And there she was, just dead, looking extremely peaceful. Unbelievably sudden and at that moment unexpected. I got the hospital to phone all the nurses and Father Phillips. Anna and Kate arranged to come over very soon. I stroked and kissed Maria and said, 'The Lord is *your* shepherd' and the rest of the Psalm. I wasn't really shaken. She'd been so like death for the past week, and it was a relief to know that she was released from her long suffering.

Anna took me back home to make phone calls to the many people and organizations involved in caring for Maria, but I couldn't then get an answer from Ludwig's number. The undertaker came to see me and we made arrangements for the cremation ... What worries me most is will the cremation service be nice enough, because we want, for Maria's sake, to make it a good one.

How strange it will be without her. What a tragedy her life was in many ways, and yet so much triumph too. The real Maria was quite special in her way, as witness the effect she had on the nurses and on all who visited her, even though they had never known her before.

12. *After Maria's Death*

5 September By the grace of God, I don't feel at all down. I'm so relieved for Maria's sake, and, inevitably, that my hard task is over. It's also a relief not having to worry as to what would happen if I became ill or died. There is – and will be more – sadness at her non-presence any more; as always with death, the awful non-existence of previous existences and the 'never-agains' – she will never again talk to her dog and doll; never again enjoy the scrapbooks and television; never again watch with shining eyes the blue tits feeding, the sunrise or the moon. But she is out of her distress and her long, hard, courageous fight is over.

There is always much to be done immediately after a death, and so it was with Maria's, starting on that afternoon of 4 September until her cremation on the 11th and the scattering of her ashes on the 20th, most of it being my responsibility. At times I found these business matters a distressing nuisance, for I was more disposed to be quiet and to reflect, but they have to be done, and done properly; and as Maria was always practical and methodical, it was appropriate. Also, at such times it can be good to have things to do and for the mind to be occupied.

Maria's (and 'my' as I think of them) nurses were all very good to me during this period. This included a splendid lunch given me by Kate. But when I came back home after it, I suddenly felt Maria's absence more acutely than at any time before; and later that day when I spoke to Anna on the phone, she said that she felt – as I did – that it didn't seem real.

The next day, however, when I was up in Maria's flat early in the morning, I saw, through her bedroom window, a quite magnificent sunrise – 'right up Maria's street', as I wrote in the diary. This helped to lift me up and I was moved to say a prayer for her spirit. Later, Sarah and I went to see Maria in the Chapel of Rest. She looked peaceful and lovely in her pink nightdress. Sarah thought she looked 'rather regal'. That, I felt, was quite an apt description, not only for Maria as she then looked, but as she had sometimes appeared in life.

On the day before the cremation, I went again to the Chapel with Anna and Ludwig and Helga. The latter two went in alone and Ludwig left with her a bunch of heather that he had brought from Germany. He was very moved. Anna and I then went in and left Maria's favourite cross and rosary with her. Anna put it carefully in her hands. It all looked so right. *Ave atque vale.*

We then strolled about and had tea, and found quite by chance a splendid picture of the exact spot where Maria wished her ashes to be scattered. It all seemed blessed in the strange way that so much has seemed to be.

11 September   The cremation is today at Weymouth. I went upstairs at 9.40 to start organizing the buffet, and Anna, Kate, Sarah and Delia arrived at 10 o'clock with food and prepared dishes, all in great style. The hearse arrived at 10.35; the few joint 'family' flowers on top of the coffin were lovely. Frances and a friend of hers, and Edith Bailey and Miss Miller came, and we got into the various cars. Father Phillips was waiting at the cremato-rium. I liked the Catholic cremation service, which I did not know. We sang the 121st and 23rd Psalms, and at the end, at my request, Father Phillips read a sentence I had recently found in an old anthology (*The Spirit of Man*):

Holy is the true light and passing wonderful, lending radi-ance to them that endured in the heat of the conflict: from Christ they inherit a home of unfading splendour, wherein they rejoice with gladness evermore.

Others at the service were Olive and Hannah, who brought her two children, which I thought was nice; Mr and Mrs Wood-house, the wardens; Mr and Mrs Harrison from the post office;

and Emma Harvey from Social Services. Quite a good muster, considering the distance . . .

We then came back to Maria's flat and had the most successful buffet, with nearly everything eaten. It was absolutely in the same vein of being blessed that has been present since she died and just up Maria's street. Everyone was very pleasant and jolly, and Ludwig and Helga were most impressed with the nurses, and rightly so . . .

So, after all these years, no more Maria at all in any earthly form. It seems impossible to grasp.

The ashes were brought to me on 18 September, to be scattered on the 20th. I had them mostly in my hall with candle, crucifix, photos of Maria and one of the Pope that she had always displayed after his visit to England, and the toy dog she used to fondle. I also took them upstairs to her sitting-room for a spell, with her two dolls in attendance. I didn't find this at all gruesome, as I had feared; it seemed perfectly in order and not in the least maudlin.

The morning of the 20th was, unfortunately, foggy, but death, I feel, is a kind of scattering into a mist behind which there is a sun; and, as Anna had said on the previous day, 'If it's fine we can scatter her free, free into the sunlight. If it's wet, we can say that all the badness of the past is washed away.' So, as it was misty, we could look upon it as we both felt and the essence of what we felt was, and is, good and true.

Frances came with Anna and me, and we picked up Kate. Frances, from her walks with Maria, knew more or less the exact spot that Maria had requested in her will. We scattered the ashes over the grass and such bits of gorse and heather and odd little wild flowers as we could see in the mist.

20 September And so Maria, *Alles ist gut. Auf wiedersehen.* God bless you. R.I.P. . . . Three weeks ago, you were there in the hospital and I would have been stroking your hand and cheek and perhaps moistening your lips. And now. So strange. So strange.

The requiem mass on 24 October was well attended and for it Anna had herself prepared the booklet of the hymns that were sung. After it, the nurses and a few friends gathered for coffee at a nearby hotel, which was a fitting completion. But not final. For we – the nurses, their husbands and Dr Kilner – have repeated that coffee gathering every year in the same hotel on the approximate anniversary of Maria's death; and we also have an annual reunion dinner around Christmas. Thus Maria lives on; and in other ways too: in – to name a few – her pictures, which are not only gracing many walls, but which, I know have inspired others to paint; in her history scrap-books, which have been kept by those who appreciated them and which have encouraged others to produce similar ones; in that splendid rose tree and in the two trees planted in her memory, which are all flourishing; in the little bird house that she designed and which is still in use; and in many good memories. [The second tree was one which Ludwig subsequently brought over from his garden and planted locally.]

Yes, Maria lives on, and she will continue to do so.

And to hell with the devil.

Postscript

As I have been asked more than once what were the degrees of difficulty for me in the various periods of Maria's illness and what effect caring for her had on me, I give below the answers to these two questions.

The degree of difficulty involved in the four periods of my caring varied. The first period, when dementia was building up, was very trying, but not as severe as it would later become.

The second period of moderate dementia was probably the most difficult, for, coupled with her increasingly irrational behaviour, Maria retained remnants of her adult authority. This combination often made it extremely difficult for me to cope on the practical level, and to endure her more unkind treatment of me. Her physical ailments were a further complication. In addition to the emotional and practical struggle of coping and enduring, it was extremely distressing to witness her suffering and continual deterioration without being able to do anything about it. Also, I was on my own, without any significant practical or moral support.

This especial hardness and distress carried over into the early weeks of the third period of her severe dementia. Those few days when, after the second fall, Maria was still at home and I was still without help or relief were quite terrible; and although somewhat different in nature, that special hardness and distress remained while she was in hospital, so very unhappy at times and deteriorating further.

The rest of the third period, when Maria was at home for the last two and a half years, was a trifle less severe for me. She had now regressed into a childlike – indeed, almost baby-like – phase, while the remnants of her adult authority had largely disappeared. Gone, too, were her paranoia, her security complex and, with them, the often hurtful or demanding element in her treatment of me. Despite all her oddities and changing moods, Maria was a much nicer person again and she had a strange new dignity. She was also, I think, happier on the whole. There were certainly many cheerful moments. It was by no means all gloom.

Moreover, and very importantly, I was no longer fighting the battle on my own. I had the support of the nurses, Social Services and others. The help of the nurses, in particular, meant that, in addition to a small part of the day, I wasn't 'on duty' during the nights. If this hadn't been the case, I don't think I would have been able to carry on. My job was still very difficult and tiring, and, at times, infuriating and distressing, but it wasn't quite the same un-happy, hopeless, exhausting and largely unrelieved struggle that it had been.

Although other carers often receive help from Social Services and other sources in terms of respite care, day centres, occasional night-time assistance and so on, and may have other family members or relatives to help share the burden, and though they may in most cases be younger than I was, I have enormous admiration for those whose caring includes the nights as well as the days. Some of them must, I am sure, be regarded as heroic. I certainly salute them.

The terminal weeks in hospital were, in a way, easier for me than any previous period. I was not having to cope directly on the practical level; and, though it was inevitably very sad to see the dying wreck that Maria had now become, it was a relief to know that she was mostly kept comfortable, free from pain and distress, and that she would soon be released from it all.

What effect did caring for Maria have on me? What, if anything, did it do for me? I feel that, in the long term, it was a blessing.

It was the continuation of a process that had begun with the death of my wife. Adjusting to that death had proved to be a far harsher and more demanding experience than I would have expected in the light of my previous experiences of the deaths of others, including those closely related to me. The harshness of the experience had, however, led me into becoming a slightly more whole person. I felt that I was beginning to be less of an elderly adolescent.

Caring for Maria continued that process. In having managed (or having been enabled to manage) to achieve what had been achieved, I had acquired a new underlying self-assurance, and something of a wider, wiser and more serene outlook on life, almost, in a sense, a new dimension of being. In retrospect, those years constituted a refining process for me; or, to put it another way, caring for Maria was a sort of chrysalis for me. I had become a little more advanced.

Useful Addresses

UK

ALZHEIMER'S DISEASE SOCIETY, Gordon House, 10 Greencoat Place, London SW1P 1PH.

PARKINSON'S DISEASE SOCIETY, 22 Upper Woburn Place, London WC1H 0RA.

AGE CONCERN, Astral House, 1268 London Road, London, SW16 4ER.

CARERS NATIONAL ASSOCIATION, 29 Chilworth Mews, London W2 3RG.

COUNSEL AND CARE, Twyman House, 16 Bonny Street, London NW1 9PG.

THE HEALTH EDUCATION AUTHORITY, Hamilton House, Mapledon Place, London WC1H 9TX.

HELP THE AGED, St James's Walk, Clerkenwell Green, London EC1R 0BE.

MENTAL HEALTH FOUNDATION, 37 Mortimer Street, London W1N 7RJ.

THE PRINCESS ROYAL TRUST FOR CARERS, 16 Byward St, Tower Hill, London EC3R 5BA.

WOMEN'S ROYAL VOLUNTARY SERVICE, 234–244 Stockwell Road, London SW9 9SP.

EUROPE

ALZHEIMER'S EUROPE, c/o ECAS, Troonstrat 98–8, B-1050, Brussels, Belgium.

USA

ALZHEIMER'S INTERNATIONAL and *ALZHEIMER'S ASSOCIATION OF THE USA*, The International Federation of Alzheimer's Disease & Related Disorders Inc., 919 North Michigan Avenue, Chicago, Illinois 60611–1676, USA. Tel: 3123 355 777.

AUSTRALIA

ALZHEIMER'S ASSOCIATION OF AUSTRALIA, PO Box 51, North Ryde, NSW 2113. Tel: (02) 878 4466.

NEW ZEALAND

ADARDS NEW ZEALAND, PO Box 2808, Christchurch, New Zealand. Tel: (03) 365 1590.